Easy   Pressure Cooker Recipes for Smart People

The Best Breakfast Recipes on a Budget

Audrey T. Pedroza

Sommario

Introduction

The Ninja Foodi multi-cooker is just one of the appliances that every person should have in their cooking area. The gadget can change 4 tiny pieces of equipment: slow-moving cooker, air fryer, pressure cooker as well as dehydrator.

This cookbook consists of several of the recipes we have actually attempted with the multi-cooker. The recipes vary from morning meal, side meals, poultry, pork, soups, fish and shellfish, desserts, and also pasta. Furthermore, we have actually compiled dozens of vegan dishes you need to attempt. We created these recipes taking into consideration beginners and that's why the food preparation treatment is methodical. Besides, the meals are tasty, enjoy analysis.

Strawberry Oat Breakfast Bars

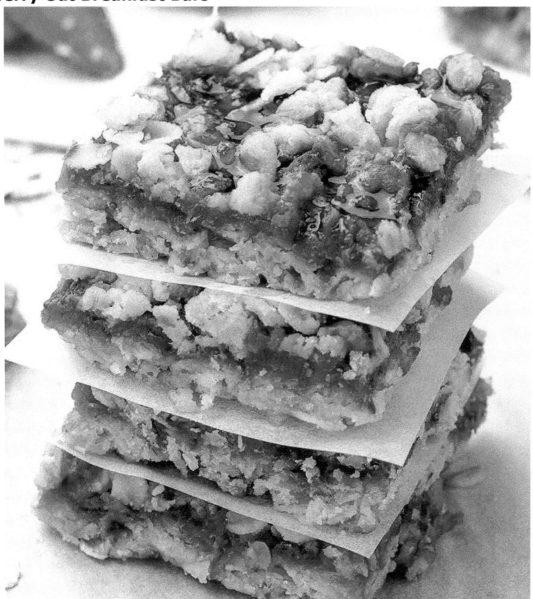

INGREDIENTS (16 Servings)

2 cups oats
¼ cup oat flour
1 cup coconut flakes, unsweetened
2 tbsp. chia seeds, ground
½ cup almonds, chopped
¼ salt
2 bananas, mashed
2 tbsp. honey
¼ cup coconut oil, melted

1 cup strawberries, chopped
1 tsp vanilla

DIRECTIONS (PREP + COOK TIME: 35 MINUTES)

Set to bake function on 350°F. Line an 8-inch baking dish with parchment paper.In a large bowl, combine dry ingredients.Stir in remaining ingredients until thoroughly combined.Press mixture into prepared pan and place in cooker. Add the tender-crisp lid and bake 25 minutes until golden brown. Let cool before slicing into 2-inch squares.

Ricotta Raspberry Breakfast Cake
INGREDIENTS (12 Servings)

Nonstick cooking spray
1 ¼ cups oat flour
½ tsp xanthan gum
¼ cup cornstarch
¼ tsp baking soda
1 ½ tsp baking powder
½ tsp salt
½ cup sugar
4 tbsp. butter, unsalted, soft
1 cup ricotta cheese, room temperature
3 eggs, room temperature, beaten
1 tsp vanilla
1 cup fresh raspberries

DIRECTIONS (PREP + COOK TIME: 50 MINUTES)
Set to bake function on 350°F. Lightly spray an 8-inch round baking pan with cooking spray. In a large bowl, combine dry ingredients.Make a well in the center and add butter, ricotta, eggs, and vanilla and mix just until combined.Gently fold in half the berries, being careful not to crush them.Pour batter into prepared pan and sprinkle remaining berries on the top. Add the tender-crisp lid and bake 40 minutes, or until a light brown and only a few moist crumbs show on a toothpick when inserted in the center.Let cool in the pan 10 minutes then transfer to a wire rack to cool completely before serving.

Cinnamon Apple Bread
INGREDIENTS (10 Servings)

Butter flavored cooking spray
½ cup coconut flour
1 ½ cup almond flour, sifted
¾ cup Stevia
1 tsp baking soda
2 tbsp. cinnamon
5 eggs
1 cup applesauce, unsweetened

DIRECTIONS (PREP + COOK TIME: 60 MINUTES)
Set to bake function on 350°F. Lightly spray a loaf pan with cooking spray.In a large bowl, combine both flours, Stevia, cinnamon, and baking soda.In a medium bowl, whisk the eggs and applesauce together. Add to dry ingredients and stir to combine.Pour into prepared pan and place in the cooker. Add the tender-crisp lid and bake 45-55 minutes, or until bread passes the toothpick test.Let cool 15 minutes, then invert onto serving plate and slice.

Quinoa Protein Bake

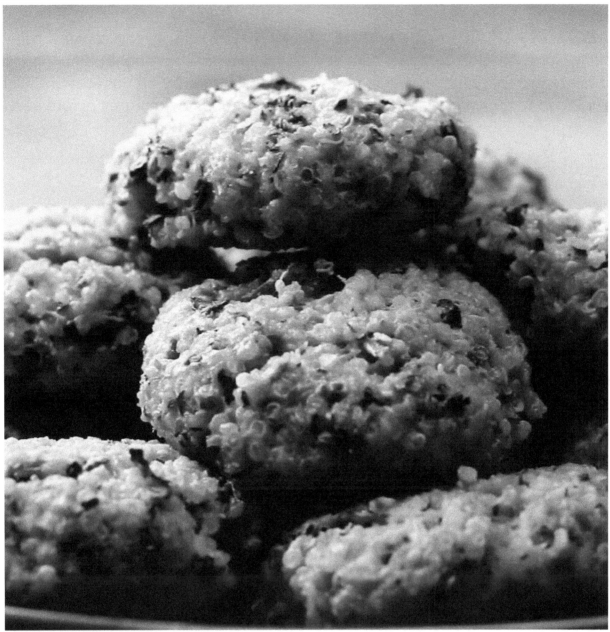

INGREDIENTS (4 Servings)

Nonstick cooking spray
1 cup white quinoa, cooked
3 egg whites, lightly beaten
½ tsp salt
¼ cup red bell pepper, chopped
 ¼ cup spinach, chopped
½ cup mozzarella cheese, grated

DIRECTIONS (PREP + COOK TIME: 35 MINUTES) Spray the cooking pot with cooking spray.In a large bowl, combine all ingredients thoroughly. Pour into pot. Add the tender-crisp lid and select air fry on 350°F. Bake 25-30 minutes until lightly browned on top and eggs are completely set.Let cool a few minutes before serving.

Pumpkin Coconut Breakfast Bake
INGREDIENTS (8 Servings)

Butter flavored cooking spray
5 eggs ½ cup coconut milk
2 cups pumpkin puree
1 banana, mashed
2 dates, pitted & chopped
1 tsp cinnamon
1 cup raspberries
¼ cup coconut, unsweetened & shredded

DIRECTIONS (PREP + COOK TIME: 1 hours and 25 MINUTES) Lightly spray an 8-inch baking dish with cooking spray.In a large bowl, whisk together eggs and milk. Whisk in pumpkin until combined.Stir in banana, dates, and cinnamon. Pour into prepared dish.Sprinkle berries over top.Place the rack in the cooking pot and place the dish on it. Add the tender-crisp lid and select bake on 350°F. Bake 20 minutes.Sprinkle coconut over the top and bake another 20-25 minutes until top is lightly browned and casserole is set. Slice and serve warm.

Delightful Beef Dishes
INGREDIENTS (2 Servings)

1/4 lb. breakfast sausage, cooked and crumbled
 4 eggs, beaten
1/2 cup cheddar cheese, shredded
1 red bell pepper, diced
1 green onion, chopped
 Cooking spray

DIRECTIONS (PREP + COOK TIME: 35 MINUTES)

Mix the eggs, sausage, cheese, onion and bell pepper. Spray a small baking pan with oil. Pour the egg mixture into the pan. Set the basket inside the Ninja Foodi. Close the crisping lid. Choose air crisp function. Cook at 360 degrees F for 20 minutes. Serving Suggestion: Sprinkle chopped green onion on top. Tip: You can also use yellow or green bell pepper to add color to the frittata.

Baked Eggs
INGREDIENTS (1 Servings)

Cooking spray
1 egg 1 tsp. dried rosemary
Salt and pepper to taste

DIRECTIONS (PREP + COOK TIME: 10 MINUTES)
 Coat a ramekin with oil. Crack the egg into the ramekin. Season with the rosemary, salt and pepper. Close the crisping lid. Set it to air crisp. Cook at 330 degrees F for 5 minutes. Serving Suggestion: Serve with toasted bread. Tip: Try using other herbs to add flavor to the egg.

Egg & Turkey Sausage Cups
INGREDIENTS (4 Servings)

8 tablespoons turkey sausage, cooked and crumbled, divided
8 tablespoons frozen spinach, chopped and divided
8 teaspoons shredded cheddar cheese, divided
4 eggs

DIRECTIONS (PREP + COOK TIME: 20 MINUTES)
Add a layer of the sausage, spinach and cheese on each muffin cup. Crack the egg open on top. Seal the crisping lid. Set it to air crisp.Cook at 330 degrees for 10 minutes. Serving

Cheesy Broccoli Quiche
INGREDIENTS (2 Servings)

1 cup water
2 cups broccoli florets
1 carrot, chopped
1 cup cheddar cheese, grated
1/4 cup Feta cheese, crumbled
 1/4 cup milk
2 eggs
1 teaspoon parsley
1 teaspoon thyme
 Salt and pepper to taste

DIRECTIONS (PREP + COOK TIME: 40 MINUTES) Pour the water inside the Ninja Foodi. Place the basket inside.Put the carrots and broccoli on the basket. Cover the pot.Set it to pressure. Cook at high pressure for 2 minutes.Release the pressure quickly. Crack the eggs into a bowl and beat.Season with the salt, pepper, parsley and thyme.Put the vegetables on a small baking pan. Layer with the cheese and pour in the beaten eggs Place on the basket.Choose air crisp function. Seal the crisping lid. Cook at 350 degrees for 20 minutes. Serving

French Toast

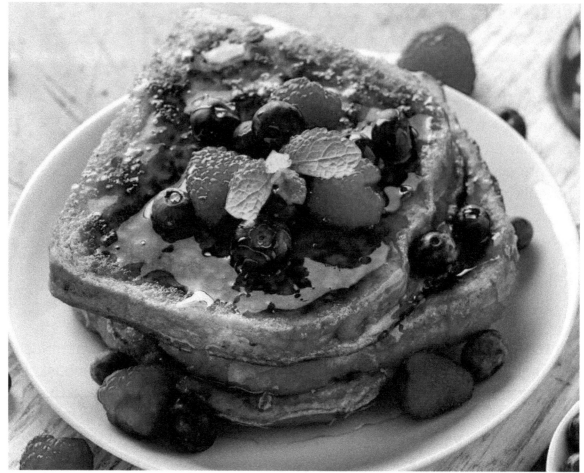

INGREDIENTS (2 Servings)

2 eggs, beaten
1/4 cup milk
1/4 cup brown sugar
1 tablespoon honey
1 teaspoon cinnamon
1/4 teaspoon nutmeg
4 slices wholemeal bread, sliced into strips

DIRECTIONS (PREP + COOK TIME: 15 MINUTES) In a bowl, combine all the ingredients except the bread. Mix well. Dip each strip in the mixture. Place the bread strips on the Ninja Foodi basket. Place basket inside the pot. Cover with the crisping lid. Set it to air crisp. Cook at 320 degrees for 10 minutes. Serving

Breakfast Casserole
INGREDIENTS (4 Servings)

Cooking spray
1 lb. hash browns
1 lb. breakfast sausage, cooked and crumbled
1 red bell pepper, diced
1 green bell pepper, diced
1 onion, diced
4 eggs
Salt and pepper to taste

DIRECTIONS (PREP + COOK TIME: 50 MINUTES) Coat a small baking pan with oil. Place the hash browns on the bottom part. Add the sausage, and then the onion and bell peppers. Place the pan on top of the Ninja Foodi basket. Put the basket inside the pot. Close the crisping lid. Set it to air crisp. Cook at 350 degrees F for 10 minutes. Open the lid. Crack the eggs on top. Cook for another 10 minutes. Season with the salt and pepper.Serving

Roasted Garlic Potatoes
INGREDIENTS (6 Servings)

2 lb. baby potatoes, sliced into wedges
2 tablespoons olive oil
2 teaspoons garlic salt

DIRECTIONS (PREP + COOK TIME: 30 MINUTES)
Toss the potatoes in olive oil and garlic salt. Add the potatoes to the Ninja Foodi basket. Seal the crisping lid. Set it to air crisp. Cook at 390 degrees F for 20 minutes. Serving

Avocado Egg
INGREDIENTS (2 Servings)

1 avocado, sliced in half and pitted
2 eggs Salt and pepper to taste
1/4 cup cheddar, shredded

DIRECTIONS (PREP + COOK TIME: 30 MINUTES)
Crack the egg into the avocado slice. Season with the salt and pepper. Put it on the Ninja Foodi basket. Seal the crisping lid. Set it to air crisp. Cook at 400 degrees F for 15 minutes. Sprinkle with the cheese 3 minutes before it is cooked. Serving

111.   The Epic Fried Eggs
INGREDIENTS (2 Servings)

 4 eggs
¼ teaspoon ground black pepper
1 teaspoon butter, melted
¾ teaspoon salt

DIRECTIONS (PREP + COOK TIME: 15 MINUTES)
Take a small egg pan and brush it with butter. Beat the eggs in the pan Sprinkle with the ground black pepper and salt. Transfer the egg pan in the pot Lower the air fryer lid. Cook the meat for 10 minutes at 350 F. Serve immediately and enjoy!

Sensational Carrot Puree
INGREDIENTS (4 Servings)

1 and a ½ pound carrots, chopped
1 tablespoon of butter at room temperature
1 tablespoon of agave nectar
¼ teaspoon of sea salt
1 cup of water

DIRECTIONS (PREP + COOK TIME: 14 MINUTES)
Clean and peel your carrots properly. Roughly chop up them into small pieces Add 1 cup of water to your Pot Place the carrots in a steamer basket and place the basket in the Ninja Foodi Lock up the lid and cook on HIGH pressure for 4 minutes. Perform a quick release Transfer the carrots to a deep bowl and use an immersion blender to blend the carrots Add butter, nectar, salt, and puree. Taste the puree and season more if needed. Enjoy!

Romantic Mustard Pork
INGREDIENTS (4 Servings)

2 tablespoons butter
2 tablespoons Dijon mustard (Keto-Friendly)
4 pork chops
Salt and pepper to taste
 1 tablespoon fresh rosemary, coarsely chopped

DIRECTIONS (PREP + COOK TIME: 40 MINUTES)
Take a bowl and add pork chops, cover with Dijon mustard and carefully sprinkle rosemary, salt, and pepper. Let it marinate for 2 hours Add butter and marinated pork chops to your Ninja Foodi pot Lock lid and cook on Low-Medium Pressure for 30 minutes Release pressure naturally over 10 minutes. Take the dish out, serve and enjoy!

Crispy Tofu And Mushrooms
INGREDIENTS (2 Servings)

8 tablespoons parmesan cheese, shredded
2 cups fresh mushrooms, chopped
2 blocks tofu, pressed and cubed
 Salt and pepper to taste
8 tablespoons butter

DIRECTIONS (PREP + COOK TIME: 20 MINUTES)
Take a bowl and mix in tofu, salt, and pepper Set your Ninja Foodi to Saute mode and add seasoned tofu, Saute for 5 minutes Add mushroom, cheese and Saute for 3 minutes. Lock crisping lid and Air Crisp for 3 minutes at 350 degrees F. Transfer to serving plate and enjoy!

Deserving Mushroom Saute

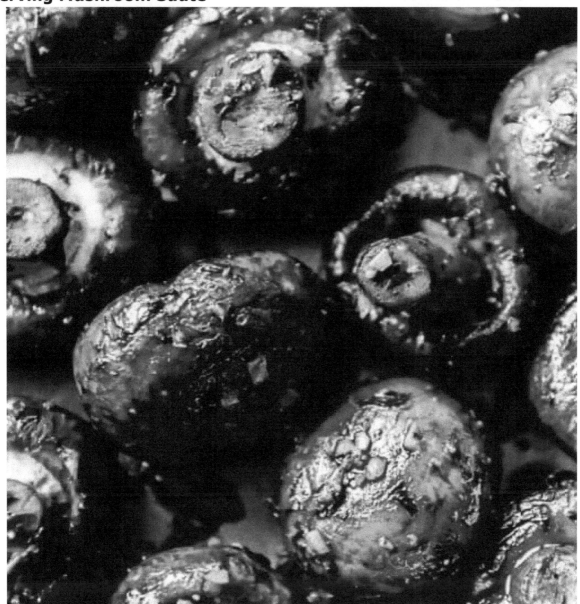

INGREDIENTS (8 Servings)

1 pound white mushrooms, stems trimmed
2 tablespoons unsalted butter
½ teaspoon salt
¼ cup of water

DIRECTIONS (PREP + COOK TIME: 25 MINUTES)

Quarter medium mushrooms and cut any large mushrooms into eight Put mushrooms, butter, and salt in your Foodi's inner pot Add water and lock pressure lid, making sure to seal the valve Cook on HIGH pressure for 5 minutes, quick release pressure once did Once done, set your pot to Saute mode on HIGH mode and bring the mix to a boil over 5 minutes until all the water evaporates Once the butter/water has evaporated, stir for 1 minute until slightly browned. Enjoy!

Bacon And Scrambled Egg

INGREDIENTS (2 Servings)
 4 strips bacon
2 whole eggs
 1 tablespoon milk
Salt and pepper to taste

DIRECTIONS (PREP + COOK TIME: 20 MINUTES)
Add bacon inside your Ninja Foodi. Lock Crisping Lid and set it to Air Crisp mode Cook for 3 minutes at 390 degrees F. Flip and cook for 2 minutes more Remove bacon and keep it on the side. Take a bowl and whisk in eggs and milk Season with salt and pepper. Set your Ninja Foodi to Saute mode Add eggs, cook until firm. Serve and enjoy!

Egg Stuffed Avocado Dish
INGREDIENTS (6 Servings)

½ tablespoon fresh lemon juice
1 medium ripe avocado, peeled, pitted and chopped
6 organic eggs, boiled, peeled and cut in half lengthwise
Salt to taste
½ cup fresh watercress, trimmed

DIRECTIONS (PREP + COOK TIME: 15 MINUTES)

Place steamer basket at the bottom of your Ninja Foodie. Add water Add watercress on the basket and lock lid Cook on HIGH pressure for 3 minutes, quick release the pressure and drain the watercress Remove egg yolks and transfer them to a bowl Add watercress, avocado, lemon juice, salt into the bowl and mash with a fork Place egg whites in a serving bowl and fill them with the watercress and avocado dish.Serve!

Place the potatoes inside the Ninja Foodi. Add the chicken stock, garlic, salt, pepper and 1/2 tablespoon butter.Seal the pot.Set it to pressure. Cook at high pressure for 8 minutes.Release the pressure naturally. Mash the potatoes and stir in the rest of the ingredients and the remaining butter. Serving

Egg in Toast

INGREDIENTS (1 Servings)
1 slice bread
1 egg
Salt and pepper to taste
Cooking spray

DIRECTIONS (PREP + COOK TIME: 15 MINUTES)
Spray a small baking pan with oil. Place the bread inside the pan. Make a hole in the middle of the bread slice. Crack open the egg and put it inside the hole. Cover the Ninja Foodi with the crisping lid. Set it to air crisp. Cook at 330 degrees for 6 minutes. Flip the toast and cook for 3 more minutes. Serving Suggestion: Sprinkle with dried rosemary on top. Tip: Aside from the salt and pepper, you can also season the egg with herbs like basil.

Breakfast Potatoes
INGREDIENTS (2 Servings)

2 potatoes, scrubbed, rinsed and diced
1 tablespoon olive oil
Salt to taste
1/4 teaspoon garlic powder

DIRECTIONS (PREP + COOK TIME: 1 hours and 10 MINUTES)
Put the potatoes in a bowl of cold water. Soak for 45 minutes. Pat the potatoes dry with paper towel. Toss in olive oil, salt and garlic powder. Put in the Ninja Foodi basket. Seal the crisping lid. Set it to air crisp. Cook at 400 degrees for 20 minutes. Flip the potatoes halfway through. Serving

Omelette
INGREDIENTS (2 Servings)

2 eggs
1/4 cup milk
1 tablespoon red bell pepper, chopped
1 slice ham, diced
 1 tablespoon mushrooms, chopped
Salt to taste
1/4 cup cheese, shredded

DIRECTIONS (PREP + COOK TIME: 15 MINUTES)
Whisk the eggs and milk in a bowl. Add the ham and vegetables. Season with the salt.Pour the mixture into a small pan. Place the pan inside the Ninja Foodi basket.Seal the crisping lid. Set it to air crisp. Cook at 350 degrees for 8 minutes.Before it is fully cooked, sprinkle the cheese on top. Coat the beef cubes with the salt and pickling spice.In a skillet over medium heat, pour in the olive oil. Serving
2 eggs
1 tablespoon milk

Salt and pepper to taste

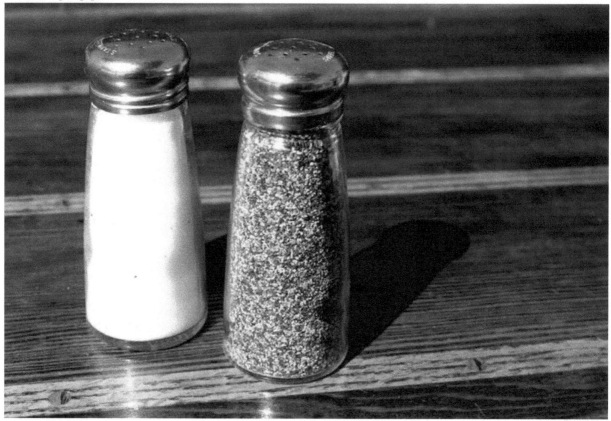

DIRECTIONS (PREP + COOK TIME: 15 MINUTES)

Place the bacon inside the Ninja Foodi. Set it to air crisp.Cover the crisping lid. Cook at 390 degrees for 3 minutes. Flip the bacon and cook for another 2 minutes. Remove the bacon and set aside. Whisk the eggs and milk in a bowl. Season with the salt and pepper. Set the Ninja Foodi to sauté. Add the eggs and cook until firm. Serving

Eggs & Veggie Burrito
INGREDIENTS (8 Servings)

3 eggs, beaten
Salt and pepper to taste
 Cooking spray
8 tortillas
2 red bell peppers, sliced into strips
1 onion, sliced thinly

DIRECTIONS (PREP + COOK TIME: 30 MINUTES)

Beat the eggs in a bowl. Season with the salt and pepper. Set aside. Choose sauté mode in the Ninja Foodi. Spray with the oil. Cook the vegetables until soft. Remove and set aside. Pour in the eggs to the pot. Cook until firm. Wrap the eggs and veggies with tortilla. Serving

Herb & Cheese Frittata
INGREDIENTS (4 Servings)

 4 eggs
1/2 cup half and half
2 tablespoons parsley, chopped
2 tablespoons chives, chopped
1/4 cup shredded cheddar cheese
Salt and pepper to taste

DIRECTIONS (PREP + COOK TIME: 25 MINUTES)
Beat the eggs in a bowl. Add the rest of the ingredients and stir well.Pour the mixture into a small baking pan. Place the pan on top of the Ninja Foodi basket. Seal the crisping lid. Set it to air crisp. Cook at 330 degrees F for 15 minutes. Serving

Tofu Scramble
INGREDIENTS (4 Servings)

2 tablespoons olive oil, divided
2 tablespoons soy sauce
1/2 cup onion, chopped
1 teaspoon turmeric
1/2 teaspoon onion powder
1/2 teaspoon garlic powder
 1 block firm tofu, sliced into cubes

DIRECTIONS (PREP + COOK TIME: 30 MINUTES)
Mix all the ingredients except the tofu. Soak the tofu in the mixture. Place the tofu
in the Ninja Foodi pot. Seal the pot. Cover with the crisping lid. Cook at 370 degrees
F for 15 minutes. Serving

Butter Melted Broccoli Florets
INGREDIENTS (4 Servings)

4 tablespoons butter
Salt and pepper to taste
2 pounds broccoli florets
1 cup whip cream

DIRECTIONS (PREP + COOK TIME: 18 MINUTES)
Arrange basket in the bottom of your Ninja Foodi and add water Place florets on top of the basket. Lock lid and cook on HIGH pressure for 5 minutes Quick release pressure and transfer florets to the pot itself Season with salt, pepper and add butter Lock crisping lid and Air Crisp on 360 degrees F 3 minutes Transfer to a serving plate. Serve and enjoy!

Gentle Keto Butter Fish

INGREDIENTS (6 Servings)

1 pound salmon fillets
2 tablespoons ginger/garlic paste
3 green chilies, chopped
 Salt and pepper to taste
¾ cup butter

DIRECTIONS (PREP + COOK TIME: 40 MINUTES)

 Season salmon fillets with ginger, garlic paste, salt, pepper Place salmon fillets to Ninja Foodi and top with green chilies and butter Lock lid and BAKE/ROAST for 30 minutes at 360 degrees F Bake for 30 minutes and enjoy!

Simple Broccoli Florets

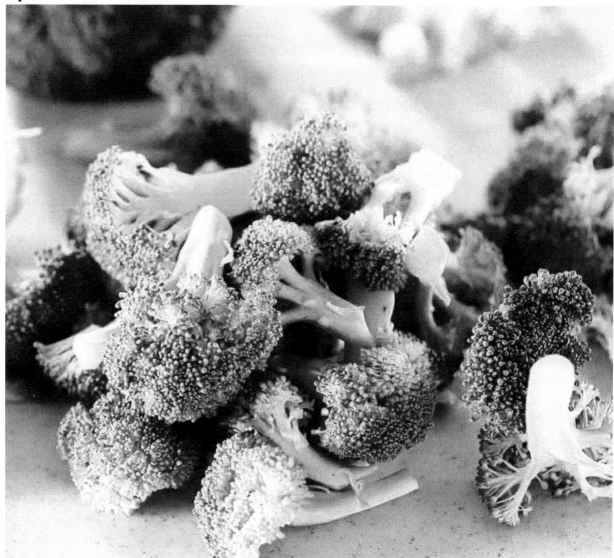

INGREDIENTS (4 Servings)

4 tablespoons butter, melted
Salt and pepper to taste
2 pounds broccoli florets
1 cup whipping cream

DIRECTIONS (PREP + COOK TIME: 16 MINUTES)
Place a steamer basket in your Ninja Foodi (bottom part) and add water Place florets on top of the basket and lock lid Cook on HIGH pressure for 5 minutes. Quick release pressure Transfer florets from the steamer basket to the pot. Add salt,

pepper, butter, and stir Lock crisping lid and cook on Air Crisp mode for 360 degrees F. Serve and enjoy!

Awesome Magical 5 Ingredient Shrimp
INGREDIENTS (4 Servings)

2 tablespoons butter
½ teaspoon smoked paprika
1 pound shrimps, peeled and deveined
Lemongrass stalks
1 red chili pepper, seeded and chopped

DIRECTIONS (PREP + COOK TIME: 25 MINUTES)
 Take a bowl and mix all of the ingredients well, except lemongrass and marinate for 1 hour Transfer to Ninja Foodi and lock lid, BAKE/ROAST for 15 minutes at 345 degrees F Once done, serve and enjoy!

Creative And Easy Lamb Roast
INGREDIENTS (6 Servings)

2 pounds lamb roast
1 cup onion soup
1 cup beef broth
Salt and pepper to taste

DIRECTIONS (PREP + COOK TIME: 70 MINUTES)

Transfer lamb roast to your Ninja Foodi pot. Add onion soup, beef broth, salt, and pepper Lock lid and cook on Medium-HIGH pressure for 55 minutes Release pressure naturally over 10 minutes. Transfer to serving bowl, serve and enjoy!

A Hearty Sausage Meal
INGREDIENTS (6 Servings)

4 whole eggs
4 sausages, cooked and sliced
2 tablespoons butter
 ½ cup mozzarella cheese, grated
½ cup cream

DIRECTIONS (PREP + COOK TIME: 30 MINUTES)

Take a bowl and mix everything Add egg mix to your Ninja Foodi, top with cheese and sausage slices Lock pressure lid and select "BAKE/ROAST" mode and cook for 20 minutes at 345 degrees F Take it out once done, serve and enjoy!

Slightly Zesty Lamb Chops
INGREDIENTS (4 Servings)

4 tablespoons butter
 3 tablespoons lemon juice
 4 lamb chops, with bone
 2 tablespoons almond flour
1 cup picante sauce

DIRECTIONS (PREP + COOK TIME: 45 MINUTES)
Coat chops with almond flour, keep them on the side Set your Ninja Foodi to Saute mode and add butter, chops Saute for 2 minutes, add picante sauce and lemon juice Lock lid and cook on HIGH pressure for 40 minutes. Release naturally and serve, enjoy!

Delicious Creamy Crepes
INGREDIENTS (4 Servings)

1 and ½ teaspoon Splenda
3 organic eggs
 3 tablespoons coconut flour
½ cup heavy cream
3 tablespoons coconut oil, melted and divided

Take a bowl and mix in 1 and ½ tablespoons coconut oil,
Splenda,
eggs,
salt and mix well

DIRECTIONS (PREP + COOK TIME: 35 MINUTES)
Add coconut flour and keep beating. Stir in heavy cream, beat well Set your Ninja
Foodi to Saute mode and add ¼ of the mixture Saute for 2 minutes on each side.
Repeat until all ingredients are used up. Enjoy

Oats Granola

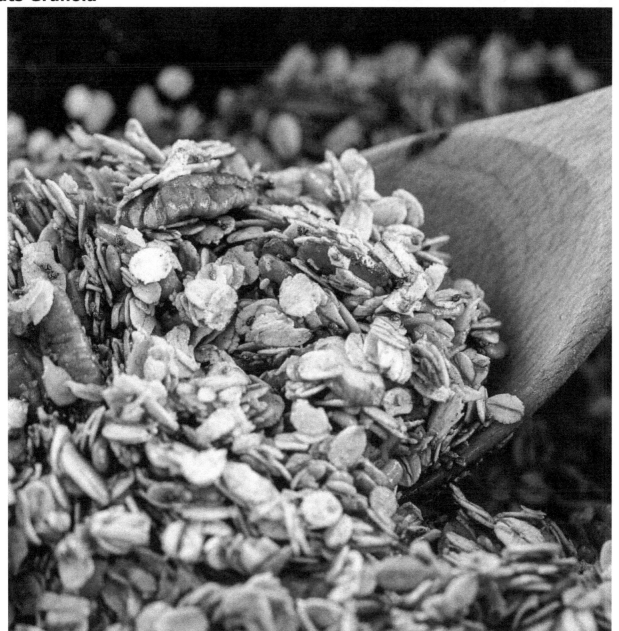

INGREDIENTS (16 Servings)

½ cup sunflower kernels
5 cups rolled oats
2 tablespoons ground flax seeds
¾ cup applesauce
¼ cup olive oil
¼ cup unsalted butter
1 teaspoon ground cinnamon

½ cup dates pitted and chopped finely
 ½ cup golden raisins

DIRECTIONS (Prep + Cook Time: 2 hours 45 minutes) Grease the pot of Ninja Foodie. In the greased pot of Ninja Foodie, add sunflower kernels, rolled oats, flax seeds, applesauce, oil, butter, and cinnamon and stir to combine. Close the Ninja Foodi with a crisping lid and select "Slow Cooker." Set on "High" for 2½ hours. Press "Start/Stop" to begin cooking. Stir the mixture after every 30 minutes. Open the lid and transfer the granola onto a large baking sheet. Add the dates and raisins and stir to combine. Set aside to cool completely before serving. You can preserve this granola in an airtight container.

Quinoa Porridge
INGREDIENTS (6 Servings)

1¼ cups water
1 cup fresh apple juice
1½ cups uncooked quinoa, rinsed
1 tablespoon honey
1 cinnamon stick
Pinch of salt

DIRECTIONS (Prep + Cook Time: 1 hours 10 minutes)
In the pot of Ninja Foodi, add all ingredients and stir to combine well. Close the Ninja Foodi with the pressure lid and place the pressure valve to "Seal" position. Select "Pressure" and set to "High" for 1 minute. Press "Start/Stop" to begin cooking. Switch the valve to "Vent" and do a "Quick" release. Open the lid, and with a fork, fluff the quinoa. Serve warm.

Spinach & Turkey Cups
INGREDIENTS (4 Servings)

1 tablespoon unsalted butter
1 pound fresh baby spinach
4 eggs
7 ounces cooked turkey, chopped
4 teaspoons unsweetened almond milk
Salt and ground black pepper, as required

DIRECTIONS (Prep + Cook Time: 40 minutes)

Select the "Sauté/Sear" setting of Ninja Foodi and place the butter into the pot. Press "Start/Stop" to begin cooking and heat for about 2-3 minutes. Add the spinach and cook for about 2-3 minutes or until just wilted. Press "Start/Stop" to stop cooking and drain the liquid completely. Transfer the spinach into a bowl and set aside to cool slightly. Arrange the "Cook & Crisp Basket" in the pot of Ninja Foodi. Close the Ninja Foodi with a crisping lid and select "Air Crisp." Set the temperature to 355 degrees F for 5 minutes. Press "Start/Stop" to begin preheating. Divide the spinach into 4 greased ramekins, followed by the turkey. Crack 1 egg into each ramekin and drizzle with almond milk. Sprinkle with salt and black pepper. After preheating, open the lid.Place the ramekins into the "Cook & Crisp Basket." Close the Ninja Foodi with a crisping lid and select "Air Crisp." Set the temperature to 355 degrees F for 20 minutes. Press "Start/Stop" to begin cooking. Open the lid and serve hot.

Banana Bread
INGREDIENTS (8 Servings)

2 cups flour
1 teaspoon baking powder
½ cup sugar
½ cup butter, softened
2 eggs
1 tablespoon vanilla extract
4 bananas, peeled and mashed

DIRECTIONS (Prep + Cook Time: 60 minutes)
Grease a 7-inch springform pan. In a bowl, mix flour and baking powder. In another bowl, add sugar, butter, and eggs and beat until creamy. Add the bananas and vanilla extract and beat until well combined. Slowly add flour mixture, 1 cup at a time, and mix until smooth. Place mixture into prepared loaf pan evenly. In the pot of Ninja Foodi, place 1 cup of water. Arrange the "Reversible Rack" in the pot of Ninja Foodi. Place the pan over the "Reversible Rack." Close the Ninja Foodi with the pressure lid and place the pressure valve to "Seal" position. Select "Pressure" and set it to "High" for 50 minutes. Press "Start/Stop" to begin cooking. Switch the valve to "Vent" and do a "Quick" release. Open the lid place the pan onto a wire rack to cool for about 10 minutes. Carefully invert bread onto the wire rack to cool completely. Cut into desired sized slices and serve.

Egg and Cheese Scramble
INGREDIENTS (2 Servings)

4 large eggs, beaten
½ tablespoon of cream cheese
½ teaspoon of olive oil
2 tablespoons of grated cheddar cheese
Salt and pepper

DIRECTIONS (PREP + COOK TIME: 8 MINUTES)
Combine the cream cheese with the beaten eggs in a bowl. Add some salt and pepper and whisk well. Grease the Foodi's base with organic olive oil. Select the sauté function, set heat to medium-high, and cook time to 3 minutes. Allow the pot to preheat for around 45 seconds. Add the egg mixture using a spatula. When the eggs are almost cooked, add the cheddar cheese and cook for a minute. Transfer your scramble to plates and serve with sausage or bacon.

Cherries Oat You
INGREDIENTS (4 Servings)

3 cups of almond milk
4 whole eggs, whisked
1 tablespoon of brown sugar
1/4 teaspoon of cinnamon powder
4 tablespoons of cream cheese
1/4 glasses of cherries, pitted and chopped
1 and 1/2 cups of rolled oats, divided

DIRECTIONS (PREP + COOK TIME: 20 MINUTES)
Combine the ingredients in a bowl and well. Pour them into the Foodi pot and close the pressure lid. Cook on high mode for 15 minutes. Release the pressure naturally for ten minutes and quick release the rest. Subdivide your cherries oat between plates and enjoy.

Sunrise Millet Pudding

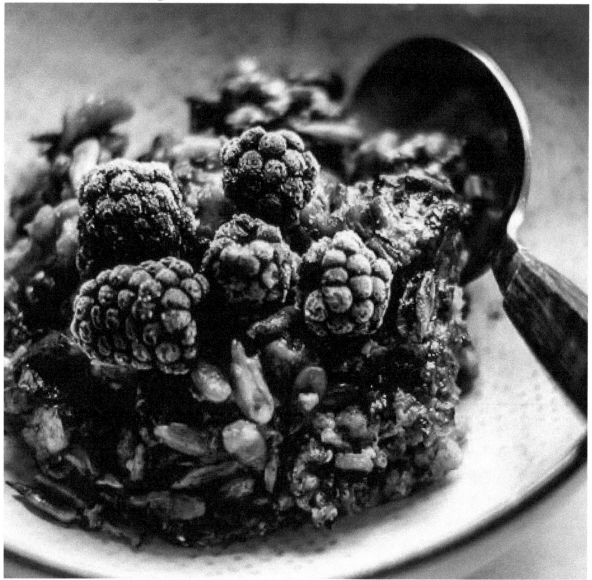

INGREDIENTS (4 Servings)

1/2 cup of water
2/3 cup of millet
1 1/2 cups of coconut milk or almond, unsweetened
4 pitted dates, chopped
1/2 teaspoon of cinnamon
1 teaspoon of pure vanilla flavoring

DIRECTIONS (PREP + COOK TIME: 17 MINUTES)

Put all the ingredients in the pot except cinnamon and the vanilla flavoring. Stir. Close the pressure lid and select pressure cook, warm, and 12 minutes cook time. Let the pressure release naturally. Open the pressure lid and add vanilla extract followed by cinnamon. Stir. Serve your pudding with chopped fruits and preferred sweetener.

Walnut Bowls
INGREDIENTS (4 Servings)

1 cup of rolled oats
A cup of walnut, chopped
1 cup of cashew milk
1/4 cup of sugar
1 tablespoon of soppy butter

DIRECTIONS (PREP + COOK TIME: 22 MINUTES)

Put all the ingredients into the Ninja Foodi. Seal the pressure lid and cook on high mode for 12 minutes. Release the pressure naturally for ten minutes and quick release the rest. Subdivide your walnut delicacy amongst bowls and enjoy.

Butter and Ham Sandwich
INGREDIENTS (2 Servings)

4 slices of bread
4 teaspoons of butter
4 ham slices
4 slices of cheddar cheese

DIRECTIONS (PREP + COOK TIME: 13 MINUTES)
Spread the butter on the bread slices and subdivide ham and cheese between two slices. Cover each of the topped slices with one slice of bread. Cut into two equal parts and place them in the Foodi basket. Close the crisping lid and select the air crisp function. Set the cooking time to 8 minutes. When the time elapses, remove the sandwiches from the basket and subdivide it between two plates. Serve for breakfast.

Crunchy Cut Oats
INGREDIENTS (3 Servings)

1/2 cup of cut oats
1 tablespoon of canola oil
2 glasses of water Salt

DIRECTIONS (PREP + COOK TIME: 7 MINUTES)

Combine all the ingredients in the Foodi and close the pressure lid. Select the pressure cook function and cook on high mode for 5 minutes. Do a 10 minutes natural release and quick release the remaining steam. Open the lid and stir for some seconds. Allow the oat breakfast sit for 5 minutes and serve with your favorite toppings and sweeteners.

Feta and Bacon Omelet
INGREDIENTS (4 Servings)

4 eggs, beaten
1/2 lb of bacon, chopped
1 tablespoon of organic olive oil
1/2 cup of corn
1 tablespoon of parsley, chopped
1 tablespoon of feta cheese, crumbled
Salt and black pepper

DIRECTIONS (PREP + COOK TIME: 20 MINUTES)
Press the sauté function and add the oil. When it heats, add the chopped bacon and stir. Let it cook 5 minutes. Add the remaining ingredients except cheese and stir well. Now, sprinkle the cheese over the mixture and close the air-frying lid. Cook the ingredients on air crisp mode for ten minutes. Serve hot.

French Fries and Cheese
INGREDIENTS (6 Servings)

1 ½ lb of Idaho potatoes, sliced thickly
6 cups of cold water
2 tablespoons of essential olive oil
4 tablespoons of butter
¼ cup of all-purpose flour
1 ¼ cups of chicken stock
2 ½ cups of beef stock
1 tablespoon of apple cider vinegar
2 tablespoon of ketchup
2 teaspoons of Worcestershire sauce
1 teaspoon of salt
½ teaspoon of ground black pepper
1 tablespoon of cornstarch
2 cups of fresh mozzarella cheese, diced

DIRECTIONS (PREP + COOK TIME: 60 MINUTES)
Soak the sliced potatoes in water for 30- 45 minutes. Insert the basket in the Foodi and close the crisping lid. Select the air crisp function and set the temperature to 390°F. Preheat the multi-cooker pot for 5 minutes. Drain the potatoes and toss with oil. Add them into the basket and air fry for 30 minutes at the same temperature. Open the crisping lid after every ten minutes and shake the basket to toss. Remove them and set aside. Preheat the pot on sauté mode for 5 minutes to melt the butter. Add the flour and stir until golden brown. Add the beef and chicken stock. Whisk until they smoothen. Add ketchup followed by Worcestershire sauce, vinegar, salt, and pepper. Let it boil for 10 minutes over low temperature.   Combine cornstarch with a tablespoon of water and add it to the sauce. Stir until it thickens. Serve your French fries with cheese and gravy.

Spinach Quiche

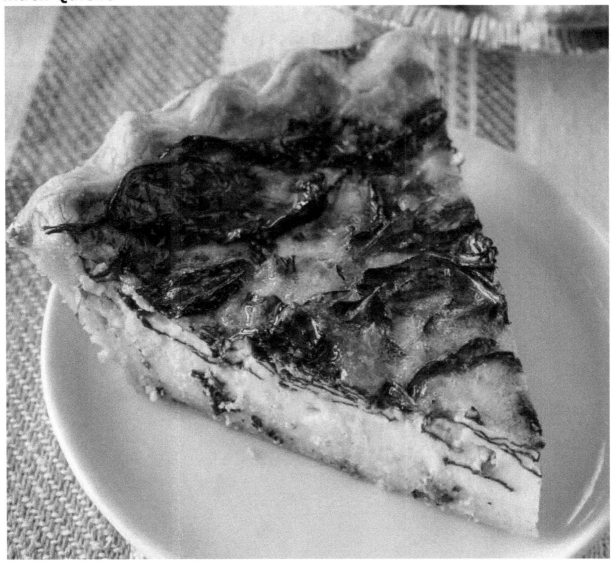

INGREDIENTS (6 Servings)

10 ounce of spinach (frozen and thawed)
1 tablespoon of butter, melted
5 whole eggs, whisk
Kosher salt
 Freshly ground black pepper
3 cups of cheddar cheese, shredded

DIRECTIONS (PREP + COOK TIME: 45 MINUTES)

Sauté the butter and spinach for 3 minutes and transfer them to a bowl. Put the melted butter into a separate bowl. Add the shredded cheese, salt, and pepper. Subdivide the mixture amongst greased molds (previously greased) and put them in the Ninja multi-cooker. Select the bake/ roast function and cook for 30 minutes at a temperature of 360°F. Remove your spinach quiche from the pot and cut them into wedges. Serve warm.

Mushroom Omelet
INGREDIENTS (4 Servings)

6 white mushrooms, sliced
1 tablespoon of organic olive oil
4 eggs, beaten
2 tablespoons of bacon, chopped
1/2 cup of coconut milk
1 tablespoon of cilantro, chopped
Salt and black pepper
Shredded mozzarella cheese

DIRECTIONS (PREP + COOK TIME: 25 MINUTES)
Press the sauté function of the Foodie multi-cooker. Add the oil and heat it. Add the onion and bacon while stirring and sauté for 5 minutes. Add the sliced mushrooms and sauté for 5 minutes. Add the remaining ingredients and stir. Close the crisping lid and set the Foodi to air crisp mode. Cook 10 minutes and serve hot.

Baked Omelet
INGREDIENTS (6 Servings)

½ cup of milk
8 eggs
Kosher salt and pepper
1 cup of cheddar cheese, shredded
1 cup of cooked ham, diced
1/3 cup of green bell pepper, diced
1/3 cup of red bell pepper, diced
½ cup of fresh chives, diced

DIRECTIONS (PREP + COOK TIME: 45 MINUTES)

Close the crisping lid and preheat the unit on bake/ roast mode for 5 minutes having set the temperature to 315°F. Combine the milk with eggs, salt, and pepper in a bowl and add the remaining ingredients. Stir. Pour the mixture into a greased baking pan (8 inches) and place it on a rack. Place the rack in the preheated pot and close the crisping lid. Bake/roast the omelet on the same temperature settings for 35 minutes. Enjoy.

Bacon and Corn Bake
INGREDIENTS (6 Servings)

4 bacon slices, chopped
1 cup of cheddar cheese, grated
½ cup of heavy cream
 2 cups of corn
4 eggs, whisked
1 yellow onion, chopped
1 tablespoon of essential olive oil
1 teaspoon of thyme, chopped
2 teaspoons of garlic, grated
Salt and pepper

DIRECTIONS (PREP + COOK TIME: 45 MINUTES)

Set your Foodi to sauté mode, add oil, and allow it heat. Add the onions and cook for two minutes. Add the chopped bacon, corn, garlic, and thyme. Stir and cook for 5 minutes. Mix the remaining ingredients in the pot and close the crisping lid. Select the bake mode and set the cooking temperature to 320°F. Cook for twenty minutes and serve.

Almond Eggs
INGREDIENTS (4 Servings)

4 eggs, whisked
1 tablespoons of essential olive oil
1 red onion, chopped
3 oz. of almond milk
2 oz. of grated cheese
Splash of Worcestershire sauce

DIRECTIONS (PREP + COOK TIME: 20 MINUTES)
Select the sauté function on your Ninja Foodi. Add the oil and heat it. Add the chopped onions and stir. Cook for 5 minutes. Combine the remaining ingredients in a bowl and pour them over the sautéed onions. Stir the contents and close the crisping lid. Select the bake function, set temperatures to 375°F, and cook time to 10 minutes. Subdivide your almond eggs between plates and enjoy.

Banana Breakfast Mix
INGREDIENTS (6 Servings)

3 bananas (peeled and sliced)
1 egg, beaten
1 and ½ cups of coconut milk
2 glasses of rolled oats
½ cup of brown sugar
1 tablespoon of baking powder
1 teaspoon of vanilla extract
1 teaspoon of cinnamon powder
Cooking spray

DIRECTIONS (PREP + COOK TIME: 20 MINUTES)
Grease the Foodi pot lightly using the cooking spray. Add all the ingredients and close the pressure lid. Cook on high mode for 15 minutes. Allow the pressure to release naturally for 10 minutes. Quick release the remaining pressure and stir. Serve hot.

Cream Cheese and Bread

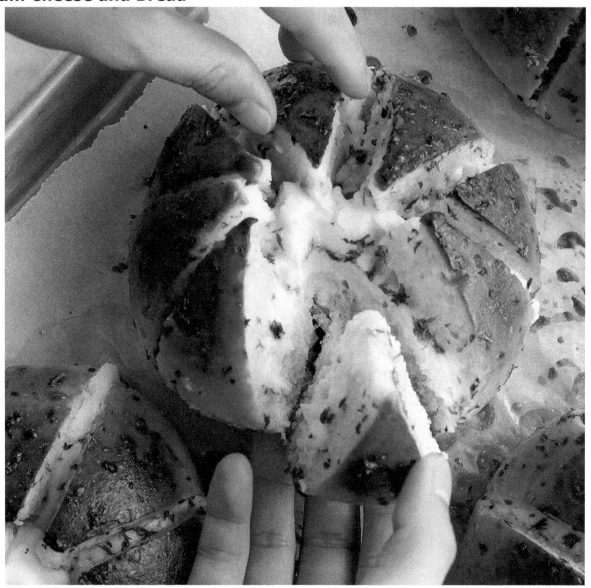

INGREDIENTS (6 Servings)

8 ounces of cream cheese
12 ounces of bread loaf, cubed
2 glasses of heavy cream
4 eggs
½ cup of brown sugar
1 teaspoon of cinnamon powder
1 teaspoon of vanilla flavoring
Cooking spray

DIRECTIONS (PREP + COOK TIME: 25 MINUTES)

Grease the baking pan with the cooking spray. Add all the ingredients and mix well. Place the reversible rack in the pot and put the rack on it. Close the crisping lid. Set the Foodi to air crisp mode and cook the ingredients over 325°F for 15 minutes. Subdivide your cheese delicacy amongst six plates.

Egg, Sausage, and Cheese Cake
INGREDIENTS (4 Servings)

8 eggs, beaten
8 oz. of breakfast sausage, chopped
3 slices of bacon, chopped
1 red bell pepper, chopped
1 green bell pepper, chopped
1 cup of green onion, chopped
1 cup of cheddar cheese, grated
1teaspoon of red chili flakes
½ cup of milk
4 bread slices,
½ inches cubed
2 cups of water
Salt and black pepper

DIRECTIONS (PREP + COOK TIME: 30 MINUTES)
Combine all the ingredients except the bread cubes and water in a bowl. Pour the egg mixture into a greased Bundt pan. Squeeze the bread cubes in the egg mixture using a spoon Pour water into the Ninja Foodi and insert the reversible rack. Place the pan on the rack and close the pressure lid. Ensure the release valve is set to seal position. Cook on high mode for 6 minutes and quick release the accumulated pressure. Slit the egg mixture using a knife and close the crisping lid. Cook on bake/roast mode for four minutes over the temperature of 380°F. Remove the egg mixture from the pan by inverting the pan over a platter. Slice the mixture and serve it alongside your preferred sauce.

Sweet Potato Eggs
INGREDIENTS (6 - 7 Servings)

2 tablespoons unsalted butter
1 yellow onion, diced
3 garlic cloves, minced
3 pounds sweet potatoes, diced
2 cups water 6 brown eggs
1 bunch scallions, sliced
1 red bell pepper, diced
1 green bell pepper, diced
2 teaspoons smoked paprika
Kosher salt
Ground black pepper

DIRECTIONS (Prep + Cook Time: 30-35 minutes)
Take Ninja Foodi multi-cooker, arrange it over a cooking platform, and open the top lid. In the pot, arrange a reversible rack and place the Crisping Basket over the rack. In the basket, add the potatoes. Seal the multi-cooker by locking it with the pressure lid; ensure to keep the pressure release valve locked/sealed. Select "PRESSURE" mode and select the "HI" pressure level. Then, set timer to 2 minutes and press "STOP/START"; it will start the cooking process by building up inside pressure. When the timer goes off, quickly release pressure by adjusting the pressure valve to the VENT. After pressure gets released, open the pressure lid. Remove the water and set aside the potatoes. In the pot, add the butter; Select the "SEAR/SAUTÉ" mode and select the "MD" pressure level. Press "STOP/START." Add the onions, garlic, bell peppers, and cook (while stirring) until they become softened for 4-5 minutes. Add the sweet potatoes, scallions, and paprika; stir-cook for 5 minutes. Season with salt and black pepper. Crack the eggs on top. Seal the multi-cooker by locking it with the crisping lid; ensure to keep the pressure release valve locked/sealed. Select the "AIR CRISP" mode and adjust the 325°F temperature level. Then, set timer to 10 minutes and press "STOP/START"; it will start the cooking process by building up inside pressure. When the timer goes off, quickly release pressure by adjusting the pressure valve to the VENT. After pressure gets released, open the Crisping Lid. Serve warm.

Onion And Mushroom Frittata
INGREDIENTS (4 Servings)

4 large eggs
¼ cup whole milk
Salt and pepper to taste
½ bell pepper, seeded and diced
½ onion, chopped
4 cremini mushrooms, sliced
½ cup shredded cheddar cheese

DIRECTIONS (Prep + Cook Time: 20 minutes)

Take a medium-sized bowl and whisk in eggs, milk and season with salt and pepper Add bell pepper, onion, mushroom, cheese and mix well Pre-heat Ninja Foodi by pressing the "BAKE" option and setting it to "400 Degrees F" and timer to 10 minutes Let it pre-heat until you hear a beep Pour Egg Mixture in the Ninja Foodi Bake Pan and spread well Transfer to Grill and lock lid, bake for 10 minutes until lightly golden Serve and enjoy!

Wholesome Mushroom Frittata
INGREDIENTS (4 Servings)

12 eggs; whisked
3 tablespoons olive oil
½ cup crème fraiche
1 cup cheddar cheese, shredded
8-ounce white mushrooms, sliced
2 leeks; chopped
1 cup water
2 tablespoons parsley; chopped
A pinch of salt and black pepper

DIRECTIONS (Prep + Cook Time: 25-30 minutes)
Take Ninja Foodi multi-cooker, arrange it over a cooking platform, and open the top lid. In the pot, add the oil; Select "SEAR/SAUTÉ" mode and select "MD: HI" pressure level. Press "STOP/START." After about 4-5 minutes, the oil will start simmering. Add the leeks, mushrooms, and cook (while stirring) until they become softened for 4-5 minutes. Add the mushrooms, stir-cook for 5 minutes. In a mixing bowl, whisk the eggs. Combine the crème Fraiche, parsley, salt, and pepper and whisk again. Add the mushroom mixture and combine again. Take a baking pan; grease it with some cooking spray, vegetable oil, or butter. Add the egg mixture in it and top with the cheese. Take Ninja Foodi multi-cooker, arrange it over a cooking platform, and open the top lid. In the pot, add water and place a reversible rack inside the pot. Place the pan over the rack. Seal the multi-cooker by locking it with the pressure lid; ensure to keep the pressure release valve locked/sealed. Select "PRESSURE" mode and select the "HI" pressure level. Then, set timer to 10 minutes and press "STOP/START"; it will start the cooking process by building up inside pressure. When the timer goes off, quickly release pressure by adjusting the pressure valve to the VENT. After pressure gets released, open the pressure lid. Serve warm.

Cheddar Tofu Breakfast
INGREDIENTS (4 Servings)

1 cup cheddar cheese, grated
2 medium onions, sliced
4 tablespoons full-fat butter
2 tofu blocks, cut into 1-inch pieces
Black pepper (ground) and salt to taste

DIRECTIONS (Prep + Cook Time: 18 minutes)

In a mixing bowl, add the tofu. Season with black pepper (ground) and salt. Combine the ingredients to mix well with each other. Take Ninja Foodi multi-cooker, arrange it over a cooking platform, and open the top lid. In the pot, add the butter; Select "SEAR/SAUTÉ" mode and select "MD: HI." pressure level. Press "STOP/START." After about 4-5 minutes, the butter will melt. Add the onions and cook (while stirring) until it becomes softened for 2-3 minutes. Add the seasoned tofu; stir-cook for 2 minutes more. Add the cheddar and gently stir the mixture. Seal the multi-cooker by locking it with the crisping lid; ensure to keep the pressure release valve locked/sealed. Select the "AIR CRISP" mode and adjust the 340°F temperature level. Then, set timer to 3 minutes and press "STOP/START"; it will start the cooking process by building up inside pressure. When the timer goes off, quick release pressure by adjusting the pressure valve to the VENT. After pressure gets released, open the crisping lid. Serve warm.

Buttermilk Omelet

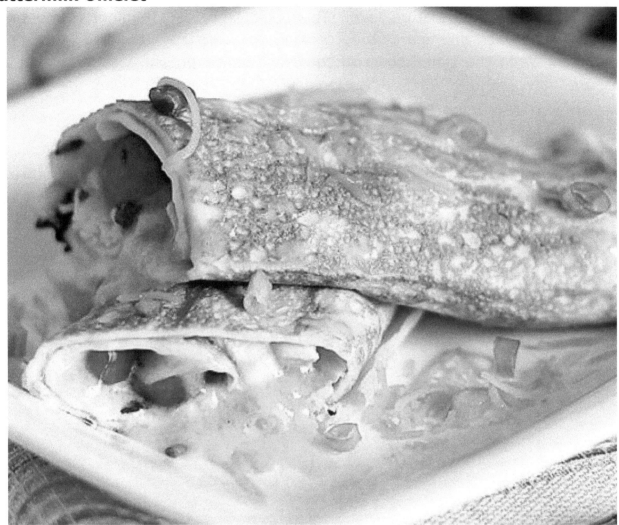

INGREDIENTS (4 Servings)

1 tablespoon basil; chopped
A pinch of black pepper (finely ground) and salt
4 eggs; whisked
1 cup buttermilk

DIRECTIONS (Prep + Cook Time: 15-20 minutes)

In a mixing bowl, mix all the ingredients and whisk well.   Take a baking pan; grease it with some cooking spray, vegetable oil, or butter. Add the mixture over it.   Take Ninja Foodi multi-cooker, arrange it over a cooking platform, and open the top lid.   In the pot, add water and place a reversible rack inside the pot. Place the pan over the rack.   Seal the multi-cooker by locking it with the Crisping Lid; ensure to keep the pressure release valve locked/sealed. Select "BAKE/ROAST" mode and adjust the 400°F temperature level. Then, set timer to 10 minutes and press "STOP/START"; it will start the cooking process by building up inside pressure. When the timer goes off, quickly release pressure by adjusting the pressure valve to the VENT. After pressure gets released, open the Crisping Lid. Serve warm.

Blackberry Cornflakes
INGREDIENTS (4 Servings)

3 cups milk
2 eggs; whisked
4 tablespoons cream cheese, whipped
1 ½ cups corn flakes
¼ cup blackberries
1 tablespoon sugar
¼ teaspoon nutmeg, ground

DIRECTIONS (Prep + Cook Time: 15-20 minutes)

In a mixing bowl, mix all the ingredients and whisk well. Take a baking pan; grease it with some cooking spray, vegetable oil, or butter. Add the mixture over it. Take Ninja Foodi multi-cooker, arrange it over a cooking platform, and open the top lid. In the pot, add water and place a reversible rack inside the pot. Place the pan over the rack. Seal the multi-cooker by locking it with the Crisping Lid; ensure to keep the pressure release valve locked/sealed. Select "BAKE/ROAST" mode and adjust the 350°F temperature level. Then, set timer to 10 minutes and press "STOP/START"; it will start the cooking process by building up inside pressure. When the timer goes off, quickly release pressure by adjusting the pressure valve to the VENT. After pressure gets released, open the Crisping Lid. Serve warm.

Tofu with Mixed Veggies
INGREDIENTS (4 Servings)

2 tablespoons of essential olive oil
1 package (16-oz) of extra-firm tofu (drained and pressed)
½ onion, sliced
½ zucchini, chopped
 ½ green bell pepper, chopped
1 cup of broccoli, chopped
1 can (14.5-oz) of diced tomatoes
½ teaspoon of dried rosemary
¼ cup of vegetable broth
1 teaspoon of dried thyme
1 pinch of dried basil
½ teaspoon of oregano
Ground black pepper
¼ cup of nutritional yeast

DIRECTIONS (PREP + COOK TIME: 32 MINUTES)

Wrap tofu in paper towels and press it for 5 minutes. Cut it into bite-size pieces. Sauté the tofu pieces until they turn light brown. Add garlic, onions and bell pepper. Let it cook for 3 minutes. Add the zucchini, tomatoes, broccoli, and herbs. Close the pressure lid and cook 4 minutes. Quick release the accumulated pressure and serve. Sprinkle each plate with black pepper and yeast.

Deli Salmon Veggies Cakes
INGREDIENTS (4 Servings)

25-oz of packed salmon flakes (steamed)
1cup of breadcrumbs
1 red onion, finely diced
1 red pepper (seeded and diced)
4 tablespoons of butter, divided
4 tablespoons of mayonnaise
2 teaspoons of Worcestershire sauce
¼ cup of parsley, chopped
1 teaspoon of garlic powder
2 teaspoons of olive oil
Salt and black pepper
3 eggs, beaten
3 large potatoes cut into chips

DIRECTIONS (PREP + COOK TIME: 35 MINUTES)
Preheat the Foodi by setting it to sauté mode. Add the oil and butter. Sauté the contents until the butter melt. Add the onions and red pepper. Let it cook for 6 minutes and turn off the sauté mode. Combine the salmon flakes with breadcrumbs, garlic powder, Worcestershire sauce, mayonnaise, parsley, salt, black pepper, sautéed red bell pepper, and onions in a bowl. Mix well using a spoon to breakdown the salmon. Form 4 patties from the mixture and add the remaining butter. Fry for 5 minutes to melt the butter while flipping. Close the crisping lid and bake/roast for 4 minutes at 320°F. Serve your cake with salad. You can also spray it with herb vinaigrette for additional flavor.

Breakfast Roll Casserole
INGREDIENTS (4 Servings)

12 eggs
1 cup of milk A crescent roll, halved
½ pound of pork sausage, cooked
Salt and Pepper

DIRECTIONS (PREP + COOK TIME: 25 MINUTES)

Mole the halved crescent rolls into balls and set aside. Cook the sausage and drain it using towels. Put all the ingredients into the Ninja Foodi except the reserved rolls. Now, add the crescent roll balls and close the pressure lid. Set the release valve to seal position and cook on high mode for 15 minutes. Release the in-built pressure naturally and open the pressure lid. Serve hot.

Turmeric Cauliflower
INGREDIENTS (4 Servings)

2 cups of cauliflower florets
1 cup of veggie stock
A handful of cilantro, chopped.
2 garlic cloves, minced.
2 tablespoons of essential olive oil
2 tablespoons of turmeric powder
 Salt and black pepper

DIRECTIONS (PREP + COOK TIME: 30 MINUTES)

Set the Foodi to Sauté mode and add oil. Heat it and add the garlic. Cook for a minute. Add all the ingredients to the pot (except the cilantro) and toss. Set your multi-cooker to baking mode and cook at 380 °F for 20 minutes.   Add the cilantro and toss. Subdivide your turmeric cauliflower amongst plates as a side dish.

Zucchini Spaghetti
INGREDIENTS (4 Servings)

3 zucchinis cut with a spiralizer
1 cup of sweet peas
1 cup of cherry tomatoes, halved
6 basil leaves, torn
1 tablespoon of extra virgin olive oil
A pinch of salt and black pepper
spaghetti
For the pesto:
1/3 cup of pine nuts
¼ cup of parmesan, grated
½ cup of extra virgin olive oil
3 cups of basil leaves
2 garlic cloves
A pinch of salt and black pepper

DIRECTIONS (PREP + COOK TIME: 10 MINUTES)

Mix ½ tablespoon of oil with 3 cups basil, garlic, pine nuts, parmesan, salt, and pepper in a blender. Pulse well. Set the Foodi to sauté mode and add the remaining oil. Heat it up.   Add the zucchini, spaghetti, peas, tomatoes, and the pesto. Toss and close the pressure lid. Cook on high mode for 5 minutes. Release the in-built pressure naturally for four minutes and quick release the rest. Open the lid and add the torn basil leaves.Toss and subdivide your zucchini spaghetti between plates as a side dish.

Brussels sprouts

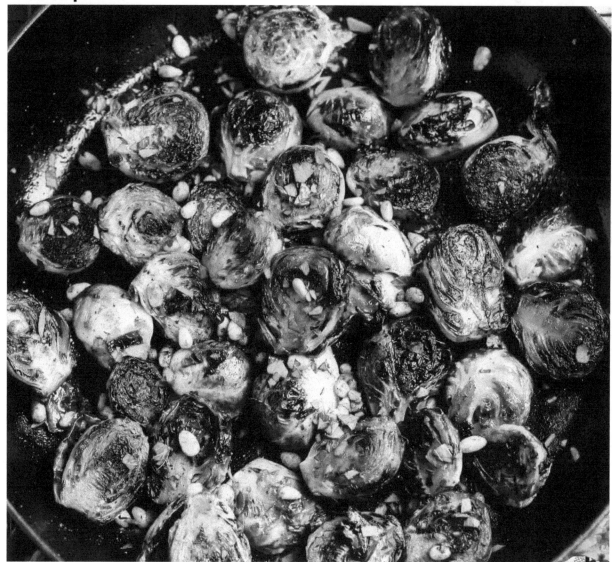

INGREDIENTS (4 Servings)

1 lb of Brussels sprouts (trimmed and halved)
2 tablespoons of garlic, minced
6 teaspoons of extra virgin olive oil
Salt and black pepper

DIRECTIONS (PREP + COOK TIME: 22 MINUTES)
Put all the ingredients into your Foodi's air crisp basket. Stir. Insert the basket into the multi-cooker and set it to air crisp mode. Cook the sprouts at 400 °F for 12 minutes. Subdivide your Brussels sprouts between plates as a side dish.

Baby Carrots
INGREDIENTS (4 Servings)

1 lb of baby carrots, trimmed
2 tablespoons of lime juice
2 teaspoons of essential olive oil
1 teaspoons of herbs de Provence

DIRECTIONS (PREP + COOK TIME: 25 MINUTES)
Put all the ingredients into a bowl and toss. Transfer them into a crisping basket and fix it in the Foodi. Add the trimmed carrots and close the crisping lid. Air-fry the mixture at 350 °F for 15 minutes. Subdivide your carrot side dish between plates.

Herbed Sweet Potatoes
INGREDIENTS (6 Servings)

3 lb of sweet potatoes, wedged
½ cup of parmesan, grated
2 garlic cloves
2 tablespoons of butter, melted
½ teaspoon of parsley, dried
¼ teaspoon of sage, dried
½ tablespoon of rosemary, dried
Salt and black pepper

DIRECTIONS (PREP + COOK TIME: 25 MINUTES)
Combine all the ingredients in the Foodi's baking dish. Toss. Insert the reversible rack in the pot and place the baking dish on it. Set the multi-cooker to baking mode and cook at 360 °F for 20 minute. Divide the sweet potatoes side dish between plates and enjoy.

Buttery Broccoli
INGREDIENTS (4 Servings)

1 broccoli head, florets separated
½ cup of chicken stock
½ cup of parmesan, grated
2 garlic cloves, minced
1 yellow onion, chopped
2 tablespoons of parsley, chopped
3 tablespoons of butter
Salt and black pepper

DIRECTIONS (PREP + COOK TIME: 35 MINUTES)
Set the Foodi to Sauté mode and add the butter. Melt it. Add onions and the garlic. Stir and cook for 5 minutes   Add the remaining ingredients (except the parsley and the parmesan) and toss. Set your Foodi to baking mode and cook at 360 °F for 20 minutes. Sprinkle it with cheese and parmesan. Toss and subdivide the buttery side dish between plates.

Red Cabbage
INGREDIENTS (2 Servings)

1 red cabbage head, shredded
1 cup of sour cream
1 red onion, chopped
4 bacons (sliced and chopped)
Salt and black pepper

DIRECTIONS (PREP + COOK TIME: 30 MINUTES) Set the Foodi to sauté mode and add the bacon. Stir and brown it for four minutes. Add onions, cabbages, salt, and pepper to the bacon. Stir and cook for four minutes.   Add the sour cream and toss well. Close the pressure lid and cook on high mode for 12 minutes. Release the pressure naturally for ten minutes. Subdivide your red cabbage between the serving plates as a side dish.

Buttery Mushrooms
INGREDIENTS (4 Servings)

1 lb of button mushrooms, halved
3 tablespoons of butter, melted
2 tablespoons of parmesan, grated
1 teaspoon of Italian seasoning
A pinch of salt and black pepper

DIRECTIONS (PREP + COOK TIME: 20 MINUTES) Set the Foodi to Sauté mode and add butter. Heat it up to melt. Add the mushrooms followed by the remaining ingredients and toss. Close the pressure cooking lid and cook on high mode for 10 minutes. Release the pressure naturally for 10 minutes. Subdivide the buttery mushroom between serving plates as a side dish.

INGREDIENTS (4 Servings)

1 cup of veggie stock
2 tablespoons of butter, melted
2 tablespoons of sour cream
1 butternut squash (peeled and cubed)
Salt and black pepper

DIRECTIONS (PREP + COOK TIME: 30 MINUTES) Mix the squash with the stock, salt, and pepper in your Foodi. Toss and close the pressure lid. Cook on high mode for twenty minutes   Release the stress naturally for 10 minutes. Mash the squash well and add butter followed by the sour cream. Whisk well and subdivide the mash between four serving plates a side dish.

Mexican Beans

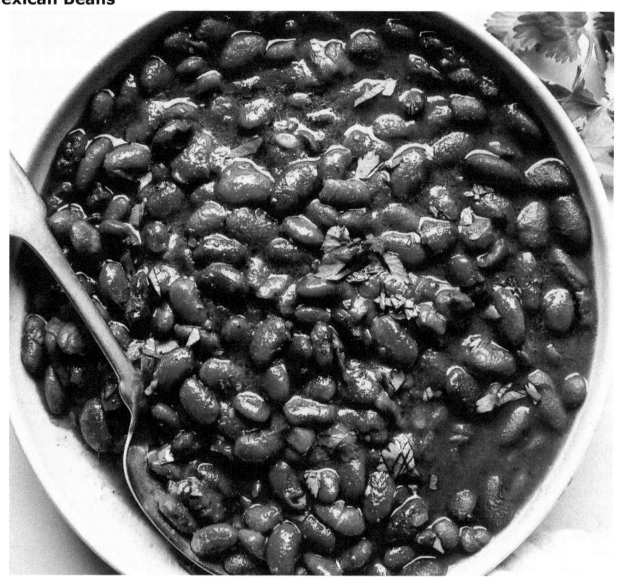

INGREDIENTS (4 Servings)

A cup of canned garbanzo beans, drained
1 cup of canned cranberry beans, drained
A cup of chicken stock
1 bunch of parsley, chopped
1 small red onion, chopped
1 garlic herb, minced
2 celery stalks, chopped
5 tablespoons of apple cider vinegar
4 tablespoons of organic olive oil
Salt and black pepper

DIRECTIONS (PREP + COOK TIME: 30 MINUTES)

Set the Foodi to sauté mode and add the oil. Heat it up and add onions and the minced garlic. Stir and sauté the seasonings for 5 minutes. Add the remaining ingredients and toss. Close the pressure lid and cook on high mode for 15 minutes. Natural-release the accumulated moisture and open the lid. Subdivide your Mexican beans between serving plates as a side dish.

Oregano Potatoes
INGREDIENTS (2 Servings)

4 gold potatoes (cut into wedges)
4 garlic cloves, minced
½ cup of water
2 tablespoons of essential olive oil
1 tablespoon of oregano, chopped
Juice extracted from a lemon
 A pinch of salt and black pepper

DIRECTIONS (PREP + COOK TIME: 35 MINUTES)

Pour water into the Foodi and insert a basket into it. Put potatoes in the basket and close the pressure lid. Cook it on low mode for four minutes. Release the pressure naturally for 10 minutes and drain the potatoes. Transfer them to a large bowl and set aside. Clean the Ninja pot and set it to sauté mode. Add oil and heat. Add the potatoes followed by the remaining ingredients and toss. Set the Foodi to roast mode and cook at 400 °F for twenty minutes. Subdivide your oregano potatoes between serving plates and enjoy.

Baked Mushrooms
INGREDIENTS (4 Servings)

1 lb of white mushrooms, halved
1 tablespoon of oregano, chopped
2 tablespoons of mozzarella cheese, grated
2 tablespoons of organic olive oil
1 tablespoon of parsley, chopped
1 tablespoon of rosemary, chopped
Salt and black pepper

DIRECTIONS (PREP + COOK TIME: 25 MINUTES)
Set the Foodi to sauté mode and add the oil. Heat it up and mix all the ingredients (except cheese.) Spread the grated cheese over the mixture and set the Foodi to baking mode. Cook the mushrooms mixture over 380 °F for 15 minutes. Subdivide your mushroom side dish between plates as a side dish

Paprika Beets
INGREDIENTS (4 Servings)

2 lbs of small beets (trimmed and halved)
1 tablespoon of olive oil
4 tablespoons of sweet paprika

DIRECTIONS (PREP + COOK TIME: 45 MINUTES)
Mix all the ingredients in a bowl. Put the beets in the crisping basket and insert it into the Foodi. Set the multi-cooker to air crisp mode and cook the beets over 380 °F for 35 minutes. Subdivide your beets between serving plates as a side dish.

Broccoli Mash
INGREDIENTS (4 Servings)

1 broccoli head (florets separated and steamed)
½ cup of veggie stock
 ½ teaspoon of turmeric powder
1 tablespoon of olive oil
A tablespoon of chives, chopped
1 tablespoon of butter, melted
Salt and black pepper

DIRECTIONS (PREP + COOK TIME: 21 MINUTES)
Set the Foodi to sauté mode and add the oil. Heat it up and add the broccoli florets. Cook them for 4 minutes. Add the remaining ingredients (except butter and chives) and close the pressure lid. Cook everything on high mode for 12 minutes.   Release the pressure naturally for ten minutes. Mash the cooked broccoli and add butter and chives. Stir your broccoli mash and subdivide it between plates.

Cumin Green Beans
INGREDIENTS (6 Servings)

1 lb of green beans, trimmed
2 garlic cloves, minced
1 tablespoon of olive oil
½ teaspoon of cumin seeds
Salt and black pepper

DIRECTIONS (PREP + COOK TIME: 20 MINUTES)
Combine all the ingredients in a bowl and toss well. Transfer the green beans mixture to a crisping basket and insert it in the Foodi. Set the appliance to air crisp mode and cook the mixture over 370 °F for 15 minutes, Subdivide the side dish between plates and enjoy.

Carrot Fries

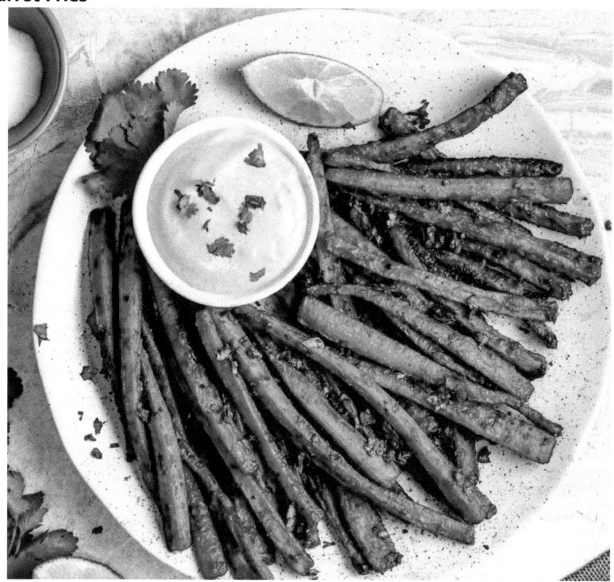

INGREDIENTS (4 Servings)

4 mixed carrots cut into sticks
2 garlic cloves, minced
2 tablespoons of rosemary, chopped
2 tablespoons of olive oil
Salt and black pepper

DIRECTIONS (PREP + COOK TIME: 25 MINUTES)

Mix all the ingredients in a bowl. Transfer the carrot mixture into an air crisp basket and fix it in the Foodi. Set the multi-cooker to air crisp mode and cook the fries over 380 °F for fifteen minutes. Subdivide your carrot fries between plates and serve as a side dish

Pumpkin Porridge
INGREDIENTS (8 Servings)

1 cup unsweetened almond milk, divided
2 pounds pumpkin, peeled and cubed into ½-inch size
6-8 drops liquid stevia
½ teaspoon ground allspice
1 tablespoon ground cinnamon
1 teaspoon ground nutmeg
¼ teaspoon ground cloves
½ cup walnuts, chopped

DIRECTIONS (Prep + Cook Time: 5 hours 15 minutes)
In the pot of Ninja Foodie, place ½ cup of almond milk and remaining ingredients and stir to combine. Close the Ninja Foodi with a crisping lid and select "Slow Cooker." Set on "Low" for 4-5 hours. Press "Start/Stop" to begin cooking. Open the lid and stir in the remaining almond milk. With a potato masher, mash the mixture completely. Divide the porridge into serving bowls evenly. Serve warm with the topping of walnuts.

Peanut Butter And Banana Chips
INGREDIENTS (4 Servings)

2 bananas, sliced into ¼ inch rounds
2 tablespoons creamy peanut butter

DIRECTIONS (Prep + Cook Time: 8 hours 10 minutes)
Take a medium-sized bowl and add banana slices with peanut butter, toss well until coated If the butter is too thick, add 1-2 tablespoons water Place banana slices flat on your Crisper Basket and arrange them in a single layer Transfer basket to your Grill Grate Pre-heat Ninja Foodi by pressing the "DEHYDRATE" option and setting it to "135 Degrees F" and timer to 15 minutes Let it pre-heat until you hear a beep Let them dehydrate until the default timer runs out Once done, store them In Air Tight container and serve when needed Enjoy!

Blistered Green Beans
INGREDIENTS (4 Servings)

1-pound green beans, trimmed
2 tablespoons vegetable oil
1 lemon, juiced
Pinch of red pepper flakes
Flaky sea salt as needed
Fresh ground black pepper as needed

DIRECTIONS (Prep + Cook Time: 15 minutes)
Take a medium-sized bowl and add green beans Pre-heat Ninja Foodi by pressing the "GRILL" option and setting it to "MAX" and timer to 10 minutes Let it pre-heat until you hear a beep Once preheated, transfer green beans to Grill Grate Lock lid and let them grill for 8-10 minutes, making sure to toss them from time to time until all sides are blustered well Squeeze lemon juice over green beans and top with red pepper flakes, season with salt and pepper.

Jalapeno Tomato Eggs
INGREDIENTS (4 Servings)

½ medium red or green bell pepper, seeded and chopped
1 medium jalapeño pepper, seeded and minced
3 tablespoons olive oil
1 small onion, chopped
2 garlic cloves, chopped
1 teaspoon kosher salt
½ teaspoon ground cumin
½ teaspoon smoked paprika
½ teaspoon red pepper flakes
¼ teaspoon ground black pepper
2 (14.5 ounce) cans diced tomatoes with their juice
4 large eggs
⅓ cup crumbled feta cheese (optional)
2 tablespoons chopped parsley

DIRECTIONS (Prep + Cook Time: 15-20 minutes)
Take Ninja Foodi multi-cooker, arrange it over a cooking platform, and open the top lid. In the pot, add the oil; Select "SEAR/SAUTÉ" mode and select "MD: HI" pressure level. Press "STOP/START." After about 4-5 minutes, the oil will start simmering. Add the onions, salt, bell pepper, jalapeño, garlic, and cook (while stirring) until they become softened and translucent for 2-3 minutes. Add the tomatoes, cumin, paprika, red pepper flakes, and black pepper. Stir gently. Seal the multi-cooker by locking it with the pressure lid; ensure to keep the pressure release valve locked/sealed. Select "PRESSURE" mode and select the "HI" pressure level. Then, set timer to 4 minutes and press "STOP/START"; it will start the cooking process by building up inside pressure. When the timer goes off, quick release pressure by adjusting the pressure valve to VENT. After pressure gets released, open the pressure lid. Gently crack the eggs over. Seal the multi-cooker by locking it with the pressure lid; ensure to keep the pressure release valve locked/sealed. Select "STEAM" mode. Then, set timer to 3 minutes. Serve with the cheese and parsley on top.

Ham Spinach Breakfast
INGREDIENTS (6 Servings)

4 cups ham, sliced
4 tablespoons butter, melted
3 pounds baby spinach
½ cup full-fat cream
Salt and black pepper to taste

DIRECTIONS (Prep + Cook Time: 20 minutes)

Take Ninja Foodi multi-cooker, arrange it over a cooking platform, and open the top lid. In the pot, add the butter; Select "SEAR/SAUTÉ" mode and select "MD: HI." pressure level. Press "STOP/START." After about 4-5 minutes, the butter will melt. Add the spinach and cook (while stirring) until it becomes softened for 2-3 minutes. Top with the cream, ham slices, black pepper (ground), and salt. Seal the multi-cooker by locking it with the crisping lid; ensure to keep the pressure release valve locked/sealed. Select "BAKE/ROAST" mode and adjust the 360°F temperature level. Then, set timer to 8 minutes and press "STOP/START"; it will start cooking process by building up inside pressure. When the timer goes off, quick release pressure by adjusting the pressure valve to the VENT. After pressure gets released, open the crisping lid. Serve warm.

Zucchini Egg Omelet
INGREDIENTS (2 Servings)

4 eggs ¼ teaspoon basil, chopped
¼ teaspoon red pepper flakes, crushed
1 teaspoon full-fat butter
1 zucchini, julienned
Salt and ground black pepper to taste preference

DIRECTIONS (Prep + Cook Time: 20-25 minutes)
Take Ninja Foodi multi-cooker, arrange it over a cooking platform, and open the top lid. In the pot, add the butter; Select "SEAR/SAUTÉ" mode and select "MD: HI." pressure level. Press "STOP/START." After about 4-5 minutes, the butter will melt. Add the zucchini and cook (while stirring) until it becomes softened for 4-5 minutes. In a mixing bowl, beat the eggs. Add the basil, red pepper flakes, salt, and black pepper; combine the ingredients to mix well with each other. Add the egg mixture over zucchini and stir the mixture. Seal the multi-cooker by locking it with the crisping lid; ensure to keep the pressure release valve locked/sealed. Select the "AIR CRISP" mode and adjust the 355°F temperature level. Then, set timer to 10 minutes and press "STOP/START"; it will start the cooking process by building up inside pressure. When the timer goes off, quick release pressure by adjusting the pressure valve to the VENT. After pressure gets released, open the crisping lid. Slice into wedges and serve warm.

Classic Butter Eggs

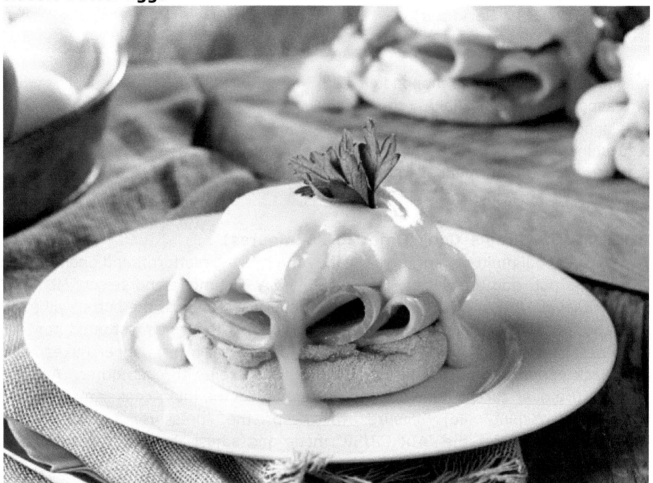

INGREDIENTS (2 Servings)

1 teaspoon butter, melted
¾ teaspoon salt
4 eggs
¼ teaspoon ground black pepper

DIRECTIONS (Prep + Cook Time: 15-20 minutes)

Take a baking pan; grease it with some butter. Beat the eggs and add in the pan. Add the melted butter on top. Season with the ground black pepper and salt. Seal the multi-cooker by locking it with the crisping lid; ensure to keep the pressure release valve locked/sealed. Select the "AIR CRISP" mode and adjust the 350°F temperature level. Then, set timer to 10 minutes and press "STOP/START"; it will start the cooking process by building up inside pressure. When the timer goes off, quick release pressure by adjusting the pressure valve to the VENT. After pressure gets released, open the crisping lid. Optionally serve with steamed broccoli, spinach, or asparagus on the side.

Breakfast Bundt Cake
INGREDIENTS (7-8 Servings)

¼ teaspoon cinnamon
¼ teaspoon sea salt
2 cups all-purpose flour
1 teaspoon baking soda
1 stick unsalted butter
2 eggs, beaten
1 teaspoon vanilla extract
3 ripe bananas, mashed
½ cup dark brown sugar
¼ cup granulated sugar
1 cup chocolate chips, semisweet

DIRECTIONS (Prep + Cook Time: 45-50 minutes)
In a mixing bowl, combine the flour, baking soda, cinnamon, and salt. In another bowl, whisk the butter, brown sugar, and granulated sugar. Add the eggs, vanilla, and bananas; stir again. Combine both the mixture and mix in the chocolate chips. Take a 7-inch Bundt pan; grease it with some cooking spray, vegetable oil, or butter. Pour the batter into the pan. Take Ninja Foodi multi-cooker, arrange it over a cooking platform, and open the top lid. In the pot, add water and place a reversible rack inside the pot. Place the pan over the rack. Seal the multi-cooker by locking it with the Crisping Lid; ensure to keep the pressure release valve locked/sealed. Select "BAKE/ROAST" mode and adjust the 325°F temperature level. Then, set timer to 30 minutes and press "STOP/START"; it will start the cooking process by building up inside pressure. When the timer goes off, quickly release pressure by adjusting the pressure valve to the VENT. After pressure gets released, open the Crisping Lid. If needed, bake for 10 more minutes. The toothpick inserted should come out clean and dry. Serve warm.

Dried Fruit Oatmeal
INGREDIENTS (8 Servings)

2 cups steel-cut oats
1/3 cup dried apricots, chopped
1/3 cup raisins
1/3 cup dried cherries
1 teaspoon ground cinnamon
4 cups milk
4 cups water
¼ teaspoon liquid stevia

DIRECTIONS (Prep + Cook Time: 8 hours 10 minutes) In the pot of Ninja Foodie, place all ingredients and stir to combine. Close the Ninja Foodi with a crisping lid and select "Slow Cooker." Set on "Low" for 6-8 hours. Press "Start/Stop" to begin cooking. Open the lid and serve warm.

Eggs in Avocado Cups
INGREDIENTS (2 Servings)

1 avocado, halved and pitted
Salt and ground black pepper, as required
2 eggs
1 tablespoon Parmesan cheese, shredded
1 teaspoon fresh chives, minced

DIRECTIONS (Prep + Cook Time: 17 minutes)
Arrange a greased square piece of foil in "Cook & Crisp Basket." Arrange the "Cook & Crisp Basket" in the pot of Ninja Foodi. Close the Ninja Foodi with a crisping lid and select "Bake/Roast." Set the temperature to 390 degrees F for 5 minutes. Press "Start/Stop" to begin preheating. Carefully scoop out about 2 teaspoons of flesh from each avocado half. Crack 1 egg in each avocado half and sprinkle with salt, black pepper, and cheese. After preheating, open the lid. Place the avocado halves into the "Cook & Crisp Basket." Close the Ninja Foodi with a crisping lid and Select "Bake/Roast." Set the temperature to 390 degrees F for 12 minutes. Press "Start/Stop" to begin cooking. Open the lid and transfer the avocado halves onto serving plates. Top with Parmesan and chives and serve.

Chicken Omelet
INGREDIENTS (2 Servings)

1 teaspoon butter
1 small yellow onion, chopped
½ jalapeño pepper, seeded and chopped
3 eggs
Salt and ground black pepper, as required
¼ cup cooked chicken, shredded

DIRECTIONS (Prep + Cook Time: 26 minutes)
Select the "Sauté/Sear" setting of Ninja Foodi and place the butter into the pot. Press "Start/Stop" to begin cooking and heat for about 2-3 minutes. Add the onion and cook for about 4-5 minutes. Add the jalapeño pepper and cook for about 1 minute. Meanwhile, in a bowl, add the eggs, salt, and black pepper and beat well. Press "Start/Stop" to stop cooking and stir in the chicken. Top with the egg mixture evenly. Close the Ninja Foodi with a crisping lid and select "Air Crisp." Set the temperature to 355 degrees F for 5 minutes. Press "Start/Stop" to begin cooking. Open the lid and transfer the omelet onto a plate. Cut into equal-sized wedges and serve hot.

Sausage & Bell Pepper Frittata

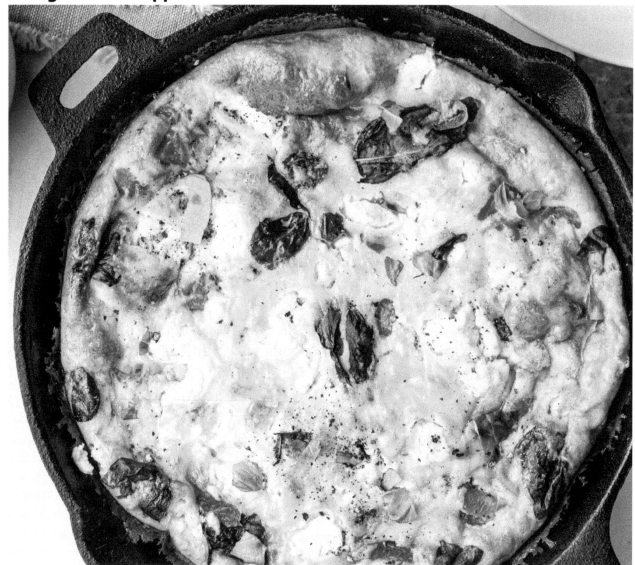

INGREDIENTS (2 Servings)

1 tablespoon olive oil
1 chorizo sausage, sliced
1½ cups bell peppers, seeded and chopped
4 large eggs
Salt and ground black pepper, as required
2 tablespoons feta cheese, crumbled
1 tablespoon fresh parsley, chopped

DIRECTIONS (Prep + Cook Time: 33 minutes) Select the "Sauté/Sear" setting of Ninja Foodi and place the butter into the pot. Press "Start/Stop" to begin cooking and heat for about 2-3 minutes. Add the sausage and bell peppers and cook for 6-8 minutes or until golden brown. Meanwhile, in a small bowl, add the eggs, salt, and black pepper and beat well. Press "Start/Stop" to stop cooking and place the eggs over the sausage mixture, followed by the cheese and parsley. Close the Ninja Foodi with a crisping lid and select "Air Crisp." Set the temperature to 355 degrees F for 10 minutes. Press "Start/Stop" to begin cooking. Open the lid and transfer the frittata onto a platter. Cut into equal-sized wedges and serve hot.

Eggs with Tomatoes
INGREDIENTS (6 Servings)

1 tablespoon olive oil
1 medium yellow onion, chopped
2 garlic cloves, minced
1 jalapeño pepper, seeded and chopped finely
2 teaspoons smoked paprika
1 teaspoon ground cumin
Salt, as required
1 (26-ounce) can diced tomatoes
6 eggs
¼ cup feta cheese, crumbled

DIRECTIONS (Prep + Cook Time: 8 hours 40 minutes) Select the "Sauté/Sear" setting of Ninja Foodi and place the butter into the pot. Press "Start/Stop" to begin cooking and heat for about 2-3 minutes. Add the onion and cook for about 3-4 minutes. Add the garlic, jalapeño, paprika, cumin, and salt and cook for about 1 minute. Press "Start/Stop" to stop cooking. Close the Ninja Foodi with a crisping lid and select "Slow Cooker." Set on "Low" for 8 hours. Press "Start/Stop" to begin cooking. Open the lid and with the back of a spoon, make 6 wells in the tomato mixture. Carefully crack 1 egg in each well. Close the Ninja Foodi with a crisping lid and select "Slow Cooker."Set on "High" for 20 minutes. Press "Start/Stop" to begin cooking. Open the lid and serve hot with the topping of cheese.

Hash Brown Casserole
INGREDIENTS (1 Servings)

3 tablespoons of organic olive oil
48 oz. of frozen hash browns
1 onion, chopped
6 eggs
1/4 cup of milk
1/2 cup of cheddar cheese, shredded
1b of ham, cubed

DIRECTIONS (PREP + COOK TIME: 35 MINUTES)

Press the sauté function and let the Ninja Foodi preheat for some minutes. Add the olive oil followed by onions and sauté them until they tenderizes. Add the hash browns and close the crisping lid. Set the Foodi to Air Crisp mode and cook for quarter-hour. Remember to open your hash brown half way. Combine the eggs with milk together in a bowl and whisk. Pour the mixture over the hash browns and cook for ten minutes. Add the cubed ham and cheese on top and allow it to rest for a minute. Serve your casserole warm.

Blueberries Breakfast Mix
INGREDIENTS (6 Servings)

2 glasses of oats
1/3 cup of brown sugar
1 teaspoon of baking powder
A teaspoon of cinnamon powder
2 cups of almond milk
2 cups of blueberries
2 tablespoons of butter
Cooking spray

DIRECTIONS (PREP + COOK TIME: 25 MINUTES)

Pour all the ingredients into a bowl and stir. Insert the reversible rack in the Foodi and place the baking pan on it. Grease it lightly with the cooking spray and add oats and blueberries. Select the bake function, set the temperature to 325°F, and cook time to 20 minutes. Transfer your blueberries mix to a bowl and ladle into serving plates. Enjoy.

Kale - Egg Frittata
INGREDIENTS (6 Servings)

11/2 cups of kale, chopped
1/4 cup of cheese, grated
6 large eggs Cooking spray
1 cup of water
2 tablespoons of heavy cream
1/2 teaspoon of nutmeg, freshly grated
Salt and pepper

DIRECTIONS (PREP + COOK TIME: 20 MINUTES)

Mix the eggs with cream, nutmeg, salt, and pepper in a bowl. Add the kale and cheese and stir to combine. Grease the cake pan lightly with cooking spray and cover the pan using an aluminum foil. Put the egg mixture in the pan. Pour some water into the pot and fix the reversible rack. Place the pan on the rack and close the lid. Press the pressure button, set the temperature to high mode, and cook time to 10 minutes. Press the start button and quick release the pressure once the set duration elapses. Subdivide your egg-frittata among six plates and enjoy.

Breakfast Quinoa
INGREDIENTS (4-6 Servings)

1 1/2 cups of quinoa, well-rinsed and drained
2 1/4 cups of broth
1 tablespoon of canola oil
2 tablespoons of maple syrup
2 teaspoons of cumin
2 teaspoons of turmeric
1/2 teaspoon of vanilla
1/4 teaspoon of ground cinnamon
Optional garnishing: chopped pecans, sliced almonds, or fresh berries

DIRECTIONS (PREP + COOK TIME: 6 MINUTES)
Add water and quinoa into the Ninja multi-cooker. Stir and add the remaining ingredients. Close the pressure lid and set the release valve to "seal". Set the cooking time to one minute at high mode. Do a 10 minute natural-pressure release and then quick release the remaining steam. Open the lid carefully and fluff the quinoa. Serve drizzled with maple and garnish with any of the toppings.

Onion Tofu Scramble

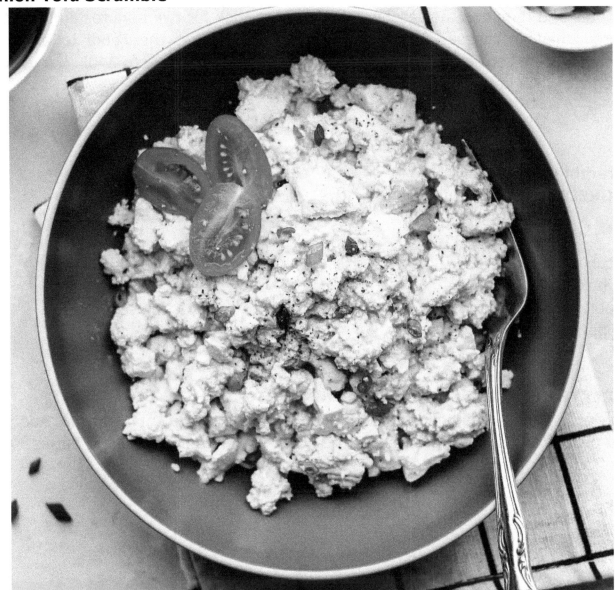

INGREDIENTS (2 Servings)

2 blocks of tofu, cubed
4 tablespoons of butter
Black pepper and salt
1 cup of cheddar cheese, grated
2 medium-sized onions, sliced

DIRECTIONS (PREP + COOK TIME: 13 MINUTES)

Combine the black pepper, salt, and tofu in a bowl. Sauté butter and onions for 3 minutes and then add the seasoned tofu. Let it cook for two minutes and add the grated cheddar cheese. Close the crisping lid and set the Foodi to air crisp mode. Set the cooking duration to 3 minutes and temperature to 340F. Serve your scramble while hot.

Scrambled Eggs
INGREDIENTS (2 Servings)

¼ cup of milk
4 whole eggs, beaten
1 tablespoon of butter
Pepper and salt

DIRECTIONS (PREP + COOK TIME: 8 MINUTES)
Whisk the eggs in the bowl and add milk. Stir the mixture until it froths. Add salt and pepper and stir again. Preheat the Foodi on Sauté and melt the butter. Add the frothed eggs and stir. Cook for 3 minutes.

Breakfast Casserole
INGREDIENTS (6 Servings)

3 cups of hash browns
1/2 lb of ground turkey-breakfast sausage
6 eggs 1/2 cup of milk
1/4 teaspoon of black pepper
1/2 teaspoon of kosher salt
1 cup of shredded Colby cheese

DIRECTIONS (PREP + COOK TIME: 30 MINUTES)

Brown the sausages on sauté mode and transfer them to a bowl. Add a cup of water to the Ninja pot and insert the reversible rack.   Combine the eggs with milk, salt and pepper in the bowl. Grease the baking dish lightly and add the hash browns. Put the browned sausages into the dish and pour the egg mix over it. Sprinkle the shredded cheese over the mixture and cover it with the aluminum foil. Place the baking dish on the rack and close the crisping lid. Choose the bake/roast function and set the temperature to 375°F. Set the cooking time to 15 minutes and remember to check its progress frequently.

Bacon Veggies Combo
INGREDIENTS (4 Servings)

4 bacon slices
1 green bell pepper, seeded and chopped
1/2 cup of Monterey jack cheese
1 tablespoon of mayonnaise, preferably avocado Sautéed corn
2 scallions, chopped

DIRECTIONS (PREP + COOK TIME: 35 MINUTES)

Place the bacon slices into the basket and put it in the pot. Add the mayonnaise on top and add corn, sweet peppers, scallions, and cheese. Close the crisping lid and select the bake/roast function. Cook with a temperature of 365F for 25 minutes. Serve your combo hot.

Polenta Breakfast
INGREDIENTS (6 Servings)

1 1/2 glasses of polenta flour
1 teaspoon of salt
5 glasses of vegetable broth

DIRECTIONS (PREP + COOK TIME: 15 MINUTES)

Boil broth and salt on sear/ sauté mode. Add the polenta flour and stir. Close the pressure lid and cook o high mode for 8 minutes. Quick release the accumulated steam and open the Foodi's lid. Whisk the polenta mixture to smoothen and transfer the meal into serving plates.

Crust-less Quiche
INGREDIENTS (2 Servings)

1/2 cup of Kalamata olives, chopped
4 eggs 1/4 cup of onions, chopped
1/2 cup of milk
1/2 cup of tomatoes, chopped
1 cup of crumbled feta cheese
1 tablespoon of basil, chopped
1 tablespoon of oregano, chopped
2 tablespoons of extra-virgin olive oil
Salt and pepper

DIRECTIONS (PREP + COOK TIME: 40 MINUTES)

Smear the multi-cooker pot with organic olive oil. Beat the eggs into a bowl and add milk. Stir well and season with pepper and salt. Add the remaining ingredients and mix thoroughly. Pour the mixture into the oiled pot and close the crisping lid. Select the Air Crisp button and cook for 30 minutes at 325°F. Cool and serve.

Coconut Scramble

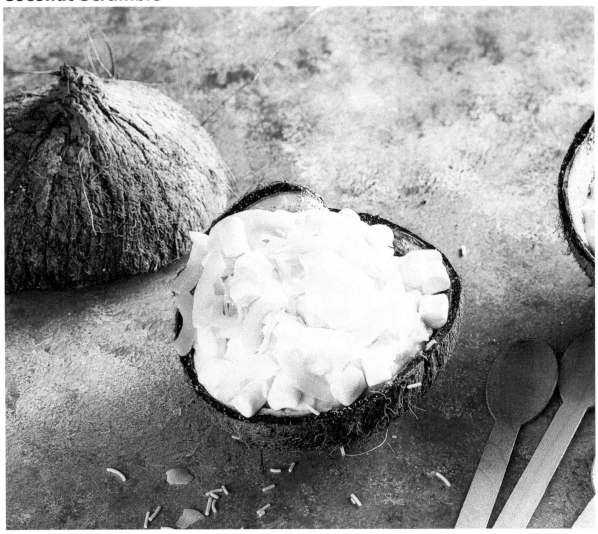

INGREDIENTS (4 Servings)

4 eggs 4 tablespoons of coconut milk
1 red onion, chopped finely
1 tablespoon of canola or coconut oil
4 tablespoons of chives
4 tablespoons of grated cheddar cheese

DIRECTIONS (PREP + COOK TIME: 25 MINUTES)
Press the sauté button on the Foodi multi-cooker. Add the oil and heat it. Add the chopped onions and stir. Sauté the contents for 3 minutes. Combine the remaining ingredients in a bowl and stir. Pour the mixture into the browned onion and

toss. Press the air crisp button and cook for 10 minutes (stir after 5 minutes of cooking.) Serve the scramble while hot.

Almond and Berries Cut Oats
INGREDIENTS (4 Servings)

1 cup of cut oats
1 ½ cups of almond milk
½ cup of water
3 tablespoons of maple syrup
1 cup of mixed berries
¼ cup almonds, sliced
1 teaspoon of vanilla flavoring

DIRECTIONS (PREP + COOK TIME: 10 MINUTES)
Combine all the ingredients and close the pressure lid. Cook them for 5 minutes. Release pressure naturally for ten minutes and quick release the remaining steam. Serve the oat breakfast while hot.

Sourdough Bread
INGREDIENTS (1 Servings)

1 ½ cups of water, divided
1 ½ teaspoons of dry yeast
1 teaspoon of sugar
1 cup of plain Greek yogurt
3 cups of all-purpose flour
2 teaspoons of kosher salt
Cooking spray

DIRECTIONS (PREP + COOK TIME: 55 MINUTES)

Add yeast and sugar to a half cup of hot water and stir. Stir the sugary water for 5 minutes or until it becomes foamy. Add flour, yoghurt, and salt to the foamy mixture and mix for 2 minutes using a high-speed mixer. Preheat the multi-cooker for a minute and set it to bake/ roast mode at 250F. Shape the dough into a ball and leave it covered (in the pot) for two hours or until it rises. Place a parchment paper on the reversible rack and grease it with the cooking spray. Transfer the risen dough to the greased paper and shape it into a ball. Cover it with a towel and set aside for 15 minutes. Subdivide the dough into 4" pieces of ½" depth approximately. Pour the remaining water into the pot and insert the rack (containing the risen dough) in the Foodi. Close the crisping lid and set the multi-cooker to roast mode. Set the temperatures to 325° F and cook time to 40 minutes. After the bread is cooked, remove it from the rack and let it rest for two hours before serving.

Cheesy Meat Oatmeal
INGREDIENTS (2 Servings)

1 beef sausage, chopped
3 oz. of salami, chopped
4 slices of chopped prosciutto
1 tablespoon of ketchup
1 cup of mozzarella cheese, grated
4 eggs
1 tablespoon of chopped onion

DIRECTIONS (PREP + COOK TIME: 22 MINUTES)

Preheat your Ninja Foodi on 300°F. Set it to Air Crisp mode. Whisk the egg in a bowl. Add the ketchup and whisk. Add the onion and stir again. Grease the Foodi basket with the cooking spray. Add the sausage and cook them for two minutes or until they turn brown. Meanwhile, mix the egg mixture with the chopped salami, mozzarella cheese, and prosciutto. Pour the mixture over the sausage and stir. Close the crisping lid and let it cook for 10 minutes. Serve your meat oatmeal hot.

Conclusion

Did you take pleasure in attempting these brand-new as well as tasty dishes?

Sadly we have come to the end of this cookbook concerning the use of the wonderful Ninja Foodi multi-cooker, which I really wish you delighted in.

To boost your health we would like to recommend you to integrate physical activity as well as a vibrant way of living in addition to adhering to these great dishes, so regarding emphasize the enhancements. we will certainly be back soon with increasingly more appealing vegetarian dishes, a big hug, see you soon.

9 781008 952003